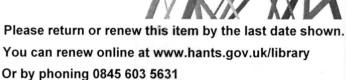
Get **more** out of libraries

Please return or renew this item by the last date shown.

You can renew online at www.hants.gov.uk/library

Or by phoning 0845 603 5631

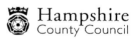
Hampshire
County Council

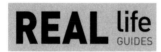
REAL life GUIDES

Practical guides for practical people.

In this increasingly sophisticated world the need for manually skilled people to build our homes, cut our hair, fix our boilers, and make our cars go is greater than ever. As things progress, so the level of training and competence required of our skilled manual workers increases. In this series of career guides from Trotman, we look in detail at what it takes to train for, get into, and be successful at a wide spectrum of practical careers.

The Real Life Guides aim to inform and inspire young people and adults alike by providing comprehensive yet hard-hitting information about what it takes to succeed in these careers.

Other titles in this series are:

The Armed Forces

Business, Administration & Finance

The Beauty Industry

Care, Welfare & Community Work

Carpentry & Cabinet Making

Catering

Childcare

Construction

Creative Industries

Electrician

Engineering Technician

Hospitality & Events Management

Information & Communications Technology (ICT)

Manufacturing & Product Design

The Motor Industry

The Police Service

Plumbing

Retailing

Sport & Active Leisure

Travel & Tourism

Working Outdoors

Working with Animals & Wildlife

Working with Young People

REAL life GUIDES

HAIRDRESSING

BELINDA BROWN

3RD EDITION

trotman **t**

Real Life Guide to Hairdressing

This third edition published in 2011 by Trotman, an imprint of Crimson Publishing, Westminster House, Kew Road, Richmond, Surrey TW9 2ND

Author of this third edition: Belinda Brown
Author of previous editions: Dee Pilgrim
© Trotman Publishing 2007, 2011

First edition published by
Trotman & Co Ltd in 2003
© Trotman & Co Ltd 2003

British Library Cataloguing Data
A catalogue record for this book is available from the British Library

ISBN: 978-1-84455-231-3

Typeset by IDSUK (DataConnection) Ltd
Printed and bound in the UK by Ashford Colour Press, Gosport, Hants

CONTENTS

ABOUT THE AUTHOR

Belinda Brown completed a postgraduate course in periodical journalism at the London College of Printing before working as an in-house writer in a number of public sector organisations. She has also written for a range of publications, including the *Daily Telegraph, Ms London* and *Weight Watchers* magazine. Belinda is a qualified careers adviser and currently works within government.

ACKNOWLEDGEMENTS

I would like to thank everyone I interviewed for this book. You were all helpful, informative and passionate about what you do. Particular thanks to David Barron for giving me your professional perspective. I'd also like to thank Habia and the Hairdressing Council, who were both excellent sources of information, and Monelle Dionne Bryce for giving up your time to answer my queries.

INTRODUCTION

If you're thinking of becoming a hairdresser, this is an exciting time to join the industry.

The profile of hairdressing has never been higher – celebrity hairdressers are always on our TV screens, appearing on everything from breakfast TV to programmes like *How to Look Good Naked*. Not only that, but no catwalk show would be complete without hairdressers to showcase new hair trends, working with clothes designers to achieve a new and co-ordinated look.

But it's not just models and performing artists who want their hair to be their crowning glory. In this day and age, increasing numbers of people – both female and male – are choosing to express themselves through their hair as much as through their clothes. We all want our hair to look good, and the vast array of hair products on the market – many launched and promoted by top names in the industry – means we've got less excuse for a 'bad hair day' than ever before.

However, products will never make hairdressers redundant, and if you're a good hairdresser you can reckon on a job for life. Habia – the UK government-appointed standards setting body for the hair and beauty sector – estimates that in 2007 consumers spent over £4 billion pounds going to hairdressers and barbers in the UK alone. Not only that,

> **"** Products will never make hairdressers redundant, and if you're a good hairdresser you can reckon on a job for life. **"**

but customers across the UK visited hairdressers 340 million times – that's almost six visits a year for every person in the UK. While the recession has undoubtedly led consumers to tighten their belts, the signs are that many people still view a good haircut as a necessity rather than a luxury – even if they're cutting back on other items.

While people want to look good, they also want to feel good when they step into a salon and part with their hard-earned cash. That's why the ability to tune into people and converse easily with anyone – whatever their background, age or social class – is so essential in this industry. If you're a good hairdresser, providing a personal service will make all the difference, and it's key to building and keeping a loyal clientele. Not only that, but professional hairdressers say time and again that one of the pleasures and privileges of working in the industry is being able to really make someone's day. You'll hear some of their voices as you read through the Real Life case studies in this book in Chapters 3, 5, 9 and 11.

> **"** . . . professional hairdressers say time and again that one of the pleasures and privileges of working in the industry is being able to really make someone's day. **"**

Let's have a look at what the other chapters in this book cover.

▶ **Chapter 1: Success story.** One of the industry's major success stories is Trevor Sorbie, and in the next chapter you'll learn about how he got where he is today and how he's using his energy and talent to help women who have lost their hair through chemotherapy. Trevor has given most of his life to hairdressing and believes passionately in maintaining high standards. In this book he passes on some expert advice about getting started in the industry.

▶ **Chapter 2: What is hairdressing?** Hairdressing is a profession that never stands still, and Chapter 2 gives an overview of the industry, charting its development from the 1960s – widely acknowledged as the pivotal decade for hairdressing as we know it – to the present day. There's also a fun quiz at the end of the chapter to keep you on your toes.

▶ **Chapter 4: What are the jobs?** Chapter 4 puts the spotlight on the range of jobs in the industry, from being part of a salon team to running your own business. While industry experts agree that you need salon experience to become a good hairdresser, did you know that you can go on to work in a hospital or even on a long-haul airline?

▶ **Chapter 6: Tools of the trade**. Chapter 6 takes a closer look at the qualities and skills you'll need to become a good hairdresser, from manual dexterity to those all-important people skills. This is an industry where you have to take time to learn the trade, so persistence and a willingness to learn are also very important.

▶ **Chapter 7: A day in the life**. The daily life of a hairdresser may seldom be dull, but it involves plenty of hard work – there's more to it than we see on our TV screens! Chapter 7 focuses on the everyday life of a hairdresser and salon owner, and you'll find other examples in the Real Life case studies throughout this book.

▶ **Chapter 8: FAQs.** 'How much will I get paid?' and 'Where will I work?' are some of the first questions people ask if they're thinking of becoming a hairdresser. You'll find answers to these questions and more in Chapter 8 – Frequently Asked Questions (FAQs).

▶ **Chapter 10: Training and qualifications.** This chapter zooms in on the qualifications and career pathways that have developed in the industry over the past 20 years. One of the most surprising things about hairdressing in the UK is that it's still not a legal requirement to be properly trained – which means that a person with no hairdressing experience or qualifications at all is free to set up a salon and work in it. Industry bodies have campaigned for years to make this practice illegal, and to stop rogue hairdressers from tarnishing the reputation of what is otherwise a bright industry. However, to progress in hairdressing these days it's essential to have the right training for the job, and this chapter will point you in the right direction.

▶ **Chapter 12: The last word.** By the time you reach this chapter you'll have a really good idea about what working in hairdressing is like, but is it really for you? Have a go at this light-hearted quiz to see if you're right for the job!

▶ **Chapter 13: Further information.** Finally, knowing who to contact can be one of the most important things when you're getting started in a career. Chapter 13 gives you the details of a range of professional institutions, awarding bodies, websites and publications.

▶ **Chapter 14: Jargon busters.** Some of the phrases you might hear in a salon explained.

You're probably already getting the picture that there's a lot more to hairdressing than meets the eye. As you read through this book, you'll learn more about the industry and will start to get an idea about whether hairdressing could be the career choice for you.

CHAPTER 1
SUCCESS STORY

Vital Stats: Trevor Sorbie

Profession:	Hairdresser
First job:	Working in his father's barber's shop aged 15
Career high point:	Being awarded an MBE

Trevor Sorbie has won a string of hairdressing awards, clocking up 42 in the course of 15 years. He's the only hairdresser to have won the British Hairdresser of the Year award four times and was the first hairdresser to receive the Member of the British Empire (MBE) from the Queen. Trevor runs three hairdressing salons and has his own line of hair products, which are exclusive to Boots.

Trevor Sorbie didn't set out to be a hairdresser – he originally wanted to be an artist. But having left school at the age of 15, he started work in his father's barber's shop in Ilford, Essex and has never looked back.

'I took to hairdressing like a duck to water and stayed in my father's shop for five years. At that point he sent me to a hairdressing school to learn the basic skills for ladies' hairdressing. The course lasted six months, and as I was leaving on the last day the principal came up to me and said he could see potential in me.

'He sent me to Vidal Sassoon's as a trainee and that was when it all started. I used to stand on the shop floor watching the top hairdressers, thinking: "This is reachable for me." I knew I could be a top stylist too if I put my head down and worked hard. Within 18 months, I was an artistic director at Sassoon's.

> 66 I knew I could be a top stylist too if I put my head down and worked hard. 99

'My big break came in 1974, when was I doing a show in Paris as part of Vidal's artistic team. He wanted us to design some new haircuts and I invented the Wedge, which captured the spirit of the times and became one of the most popular cuts of the decade. Achieving that made me think: "If I can do this once, I can do it again."'

Five years later, when he was working at John Frieda as a top stylist, Trevor invented scrunch drying. This method of drying, which adds volume and texture to the hair, caught on across the world and helped to make him a household name.

It wasn't long afterwards that a man called Grant Peet, whom he'd met on the hairdressing circuit, contacted him to ask if he'd like to run his salon in Russell Street, Covent Garden.

'I said yes, if I could have 50% and my name over the door. I was there for 20 years and moved to my present salon in Floral Street 10 years ago because we couldn't fit enough people into the Russell Street salon.

'I now have 46 employees in the London salon, about 25 in my Brighton salon and 12 in my Manchester salon, which is new. I work in all three; I'm there to ensure that standards are kept up. At the end of the day, the only difference between one hairdresser and another is in the quality of work.

'All my trainees undertake a training course that's exclusive to my company. It takes an average of three years to complete and they have to pass nine tests before they can become a stylist. I oversee the final test; no one works on the floor without my approval. Out of 10 people I employ from scratch, a maximum of two will make it. I will not drop my standards.

'I believe that qualifications for hairdressers should be mandatory in this country. We're working with sharp implements and with chemicals that can burn, and we need a level of standards across the industry.

'To succeed in hairdressing, you have to enjoy being with people. You're dealing with people from all walks of life and you've got to be able to hold a conversation with them. You also need stamina: you're on your feet all day and you might not get a lunch hour if you overrun. It's hard work and it's physically demanding.

'Over the past 10 to 15 years, hairdressing has been glamorised in TV programmes and on fashion shows. Whether I like it or not, I'm known as a celebrity hairdresser, and the idea of becoming a celebrity is very attractive to young people.

> 66 To succeed in hairdressing, you have to enjoy being with people. 99

'But Michael Schumacher didn't become a world champion the day after his driving test and it's the same in this industry: it doesn't happen overnight. Some young people don't want to take time to do their Apprenticeship because they want it all tomorrow. But you've got to be prepared to put in the hard work on the front end before you can receive any rewards.

'If you seriously want to be a hairdresser, go to the best salon in your area – the one that offers in-house training. The reason it will be the best is because it has a higher standard and quality of work. It will teach you good habits rather than bad ones and it can be a springboard to other things.

'You can learn skills in a college, but hairdressing takes place in a salon, and you have to work in a salon to understand the busyness and the pressures. It's all part of the learning.'

Another major turning point for Trevor was when his sister-in-law became ill with cancer five years ago. 'She knew she'd lose her hair because of the treatment and asked me to get a wig for her. I found one and cut it on her because it looked like a wig before I started. When she saw herself in the mirror she burst into tears, and they were tears of joy.

'That's when the penny dropped for me. When I cut people's hair in a salon, they liked it but they never burst into tears. I wanted to do more to help the people who really needed it.'

Trevor set up a registered charity called My New Hair, which works with the NHS to improve the quality of wigs available to patients.

'Being told she has cancer and will lose her hair is devastating news for any woman. She doesn't know what to do or where to go. I want to change that by making information packs available in doctors' surgeries and hospitals.

'I've already trained around 200 hairdressers to customise wigs – cutting wigs to suit a particular person. My goal is to train 400; if I do that, L'Oréal will take the whole idea internationally.

'My goals have changed over the years and this is the most satisfying thing I've ever done. I attend conferences and give talks about this work, both in this country and abroad. Throughout my career I've been involved with hair shows and fashion seminars, but I'm handing that work over to my creative director.

'I've stopped cutting hair in my salons so I can concentrate on my work for cancer patients. I could earn £10,000 a week cutting clients' hair but I'm doing this work for nothing.

'I still find hairdressing really exciting – it can give you so much satisfaction. Now is a great time to start a career in the industry because there are so many options. You can work in a salon, you can be a session hairdresser for magazines or TV commercials, you can teach hairdressing and travel the world. Hairdressing has really spread its wings over the past 20 years.

> 66 Now is a great time to start a career in the industry because there are so many options. 99

'I've made it my life and I don't regret that.'

CHAPTER 2
WHAT IS HAIRDRESSING?

As you've probably gathered already, hairdressing is a popular and versatile service industry that can earn you a good living and open the door to exciting opportunities.

Hairdressing is a strong industry, employing over 190,000 people across the UK and with more than half that number in training. Salons range from small enterprises (businesses) – the vast majority in the UK are private set-ups employing fewer then 10 people – to large national chains.

Together, these three industries comprise the hair sector:

1. hairdressing
2. barbering
3. African-type hairdressing and barbering.

Most salons cater for the whole range of clients, although barbers' shops and African-type salons are geared to specific clientele. These days there's a high proportion of unisex salons serving both men and women, meaning that traditional barbers' shops – which serve mainly men – have a smaller slice of the market than they once did.

While African-type salons may be relatively small in number, they're a thriving part of the industry. Unlike salons in general, which are spread across the UK, they tend to be concentrated in city areas. They specialise in techniques like plaiting, braiding, attaching hair extensions, chemical relaxing and natural (non-chemical) hairdressing.

A SNIPPET OF HISTORY

Over the past few decades, hairdressing has gone from strength to strength. While even a casual stroll through recent history will reveal a wealth of trends, from the fingerwaving of the 1920s and 1930s to the bouffant styles that started life in the 1950s, the 1960s was a major turning point for hairdressing as we know it today.

This was an era of social unrest and change, with young people challenging convention in every area of their lives. Pop groups such as the Beatles revolutionised music, designers such as Mary Quant pushed forward the frontiers of fashion and hairdressers such as Vidal Sassoon changed the face of hairdressing.

LEARN THE LINGO
Don't know what a word means? Turn to the Jargon Busters chapter on page 101 to find out.

Sassoon's simple and precise cutting techniques ushered in a new era for the industry and formed the foundation for modern hairdressing. He turned established convention on its head by dispensing with hairpins and rollers and cutting hair to suit a client's face shape and bone structure. Like other hairdressers who followed in his wake, Sassoon made his name by creating new haircuts for women, who were increasingly looking for styles that were easy to maintain.

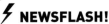 **NEWSFLASH!**

One of Vidal Sassoon's most famous cuts was the geometrically styled five point cut. He was also one of the first hairdressers to lend his name to a line of hair care products and a salon chain.

By the late 1960s, unisex hairdressing had come into fashion. Barbers had to adapt to longer hairstyles for men and it became acceptable for a man to step into a salon for a haircut – another trend that has continued into the present day. The decade also saw the passing of the Hairdressers (Registration) Act in 1964. This led to the creation of the Hairdressing Council, which set up a register of qualified hairdressers. Hairdressers could now apply to become state registered, which gave them official recognition in the public eye.

THE IMPORTANCE OF REGISTRATION

Surprisingly in such a high-profile industry, registration in the UK is still only voluntary. As we said in the Introduction, anyone can legally set up and practise as a hairdresser, even without qualifications or training (which are now rigorous in most parts of the industry). The Hairdressing Council, along with other bodies in the industry, continues to campaign for registration to be a legal requirement. This would help

TOP TIP!

You can find out more on www.haircouncil.org.uk.

weed out those cowboy (or cowgirl) hairdressers who give the industry a bad name by delivering a sub-standard service.

Sally Styles, Registrar of the Hairdressing Council, says the UK is out of step with Europe – and most of the world – in not making qualifications mandatory: 'Hairdressing requires high levels of technical skill and the ability to work safely with powerful chemicals, so we need mandatory rules and regulations to protect both consumers and the reputation of the industry.'

BECOMING A STATE REGISTERED HAIRDRESSER (SRH)

This makes you part of a group of registered professionals – like doctors, dentists and physiotherapists. You can become an SRH after you've achieved NVQ level 2 in Hairdressing or its equivalent. The benefits include:

- ▶ a certificate showing that you are recognised as a hairdresser under the Hairdressers (Registration) Act
- ▶ the right to use the initials SRH after your name
- ▶ your name on the Hairdressing Council website, which contains the only listing of officially recognised stylists in the UK
- ▶ the right to apply for the Master Craftsman's Diploma, possibly after two years of registration
- ▶ useful (and sometimes necessary) credentials to practise hairdressing in Europe, America and elsewhere
- ▶ access to free advice, competitively priced insurance cover and the widely read *Hairdresser* magazine, all through the Hairdressing Council

- ▶ access to SRH promotional items
- ▶ the opportunity to attend receptions in Parliament and meet politicians and top names in the hairdressing industry.

THE INDUSTRY TODAY

These days, if you gain the right qualifications and are prepared to work hard, the rewards can be very good. There's a whole range of opportunities on offer, from competitions sponsored by major product companies to seminars where you can learn from big names in the industry.

Gone are the days when people fell into hairdressing because they didn't make any headway at school. It's now a competitive and sophisticated profession with clearly defined progression routes.

The recognised qualification across the industry is the National Vocational Qualification (NVQ), or Scottish Vocational Qualification (SVQ) in Scotland. There is also the Diploma in Hair and Beauty Studies, which is another route into the industry.

Over 80% of hairdressers and barbers have achieved a qualification relevant to the industry and more than 60% are qualified to NVQ level 2, which compares favourably with skills levels across the economy. However, the emphasis these days is on upskilling, and the industry standard is now NVQ level 3. A number of salons help employees attain NVQs through in-house training schemes or Apprenticeships (you can read more about these in Chapter 10).

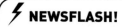

NEWSFLASH!

At present, over 50% of hairdressers are aged 34 or younger.

Although you can become a hairdresser at any age, hairdressing is a young industry which has always relied heavily on entrants under the age of 24. This may change as young people stay in education for longer and the general population becomes older, which will mean decreasing numbers of young people entering the workforce. (The industry already employs a high proportion of workers from abroad, especially in major cities such as London.)

However, one of the hallmarks of hairdressing is its flexibility. Many people return to the industry after having a family, often on a freelance or part-time basis, and over 40% of hairdressers are self-employed.

Sheila Abrahams, a Director of the Freelance Hair and Beauty Federation (FHBF), the only trade body for self-employed people in the industry. She helped to set up the FHBF in 1993 to promote the professional interests of freelance hair stylists and beauty therapists.

66 Being freelance isn't as easy as people may think – you're out on your own and don't have colleagues to back you up. **99**

'We set a standard across the industry – our members must be qualified and experienced and must have public liability insurance. We encourage them to set up a proper business and charge realistic prices; there's a common misconception that freelances will provide a service on the cheap, but they're the same calibre as salon stylists and deserve the same rewards. Being freelance isn't as easy as people may think – you're out on your own and don't have colleagues to back you up. That's why it's so important to gain salon experience before going freelance. I'd say two years is an absolute minimum.'

Hairdressing has always been a female-dominated industry – in 2007, it was 90% female and 10% male. However, Sheila for one is observing more male entrants approach it as a serious profession.

'When I started out in the industry, men often didn't stay long; hairdressing was something they did until they could find a better job. That's changing as they see the example set by mature male icons who have made a name for themselves in the industry. It's an exciting time to be in hairdressing.

❝ In hairdressing, you never stop learning and that's part of the fascination. ❞

'For me, hairdressing has always been a passion. I studied it at college, worked in a salon, owned a salon, had a family and then went freelance. In all that time, there hasn't been one day when I've got up and not wanted to go to work. In hairdressing, you never stop learning and that's part of the fascination.'

AN EXCITING INDUSTRY TO BUILD YOUR CAREER IN

Sheila's experience is far from unique. According to the annual City & Guilds Happiness Index, hairdressers are the happiest workers of all. Like beauty therapists, who

⚡ NEWSFLASH!

The Happiness Index surveys a sample of UK workers across a range of professions to gauge how contented they are at work. For five consecutive years hairdressers ranked in the top two positions every year except one, when they were overtaken by disc jockeys!

also ranked highly, hairdressers said that strong relationships with their colleagues and feeling valued for what they did made all the difference. They also felt motivated by a genuine interest in their work and by having access to good training and development opportunities.

As the industry continues to move forward, the range of services on offer is likely to keep expanding. These days, it's increasingly common for salons to offer beauty treatments such as manicures and massage, as well as to actively promote new products coming on to the market. That means it's important for anyone working in the industry to keep up to date with trends and developments.

> **❝** It takes years rather than months to become a good hairdresser, and industry experts stress the importance of learning to walk before you can run. **❞**

There's a continuing demand for good stylists, as well as skills gaps in specific areas, including African-type hairdressing, long hair dressing, hair extensions, colour correction and traditional barbering skills. While this is encouraging for prospective entrants, it's important to remember that you won't gain any of those skills overnight. It takes years rather than months to become a good hairdresser, and industry experts stress the importance of learning to walk before you can run.

Once you've learned the ropes and proved you've got what it takes to succeed, hairdressing can open up a host of opportunities, from joining a salon art team to becoming a college lecturer.

HAIRDRESSING QUIZ

By now you're probably getting a good idea of what hairdressing is about, and you'll have seen how it's evolved into the fast-moving and exciting industry it is today. To discover how much you've learned, take a few moments to answer the multiple choice quiz below. You might be surprised to discover how much you already know.

1 **What is the UK government-appointed body that sets standards for the hair and beauty sector?**
A. The Hairdressing Council
B. Habia
C. The Freelance Hair and Beauty Federation

2 **The vast majority of hairdressing salons are:**
A. Individual outlets
B. Public enterprises
C. Large chains

3 **How long should you work in a salon before going freelance?**
A. Six months
B. A year
C. At least two years

4 **What made Vidal Sassoon famous?**
A. The bouffant hairstyle
B. His simple and precise cutting techniques
C. The blue rinse

5 **What did the passing of the 1964 Hairdressers (Registration) Act achieve?**

A. It led to the creation of the Hairdressing Council, which set up a voluntary register of qualified hairdressers

B. It made it a legal requirement to be fully qualified before you could practise as a hairdresser

C. It legalised unisex hairstyles

6 **Well-defined routes to different careers in hairdressing have developed over the past:**

A. 50 years

B. 20 years

C. Five years

7 **What proportion of hairdressers are self-employed?**

A. 15%

B. 80%

C. Over 40%

8 **What's the gender balance like in the industry?**

A. There are more women than men

B. There are more men than women

C. There's an even balance between the sexes

9 **A City & Guilds Happiness Index surveys have found that:**

A. Most hairdressers are put off by the hard work and long hours

B. Hairdressers are the happiest workers

C. Hairdressers tend to be demotivated

10 **To be a good hairdresser, you need:**

A. A genuine interest in people

B. Good technical skills

C. Plenty of enthusiasm

ANSWERS

1 **B** – Habia creates the standards that form the basis of all hairdressing qualifications, as well as industry codes of practice. It also provides advice on a range of matters including careers, business development and salon safety. You can find out more at www.habia.org.

2 **A** – Around 85% of salons are individual outlets where the manager works alongside the employees. Around 15% are salon chains, often with three or four outlets. Large chains and franchises such as Regis and Toni & Guy represent only about 2% of hairdressing outlets. Around 99% of hair and beauty sector establishments are private enterprises.

3 **C** – The Freelance Hair and Beauty Federation (FHBF) requires its members to have at least two years' salon experience, preferably more. Seasoned hairdressers stress that working in a salon is an essential part of learning to become a hairdresser, enabling you to experience the business at first hand and learn from professionals on the job.

4 **B** – Vidal Sassoon built his reputation on simple, precise haircuts at a time when back-combed and heavily lacquered hairstyles were in vogue. These declined in popularity and Sassoon's revolutionary approach became the foundation for modern hairdressing. Many of the haircuts he created are still popular today.

The blue rinse is a dilute hair dye which gives greying or yellow-white hair a bluish tinge. It has declined in popularity since the 1940s and 1950s.

5 **A** – Although the Act enabled hairdressers to become state registered, this was only voluntary and it's still not illegal to practise as a hairdresser without being properly trained. The Hairdressing Council, which maintains the state register, campaigns for registration to become a legal requirement. You can find out more at www.haircouncil.org.uk.

6 **B** – Although career routes and qualifications in hairdressing have continued to evolve over the past five years, the current system of Apprenticeships, training and structured career pathways has developed over the past 20 years. Before that it wasn't the norm to receive formal training, and people learned the trade on the job.

7 **C** – Over 40% of hairdressers are self-employed, mostly on a freelance basis but also as salon owners. Some choose to 'mix and match' self-employment and employment – working part time in a salon and part time for themselves. One of the beauties of hairdressing is the flexibility if offers to go freelance. You can find out more from the Freelance Hair and Beauty Federation website: www.fhbf.org.uk.

8 **A** – Hairdressing is a heavily female-dominated industry. However, a high proportion of leading hairdressers are men, who serve as role models for younger men coming into the industry.

9 **B** – Hairdressers have scored consistently highly in Happiness Index surveys, citing good relationships with their colleagues and being valued for what they do as major reasons for enjoying the job. (You can find out more at www.cityandguilds.com/happiness.)

10 This is a trick question: the answer is all three! Hairdressing is a service industry where it's essential to be interested in people and to have good communication skills. But it's also a practical trade that requires good technical skills and attention to detail. And to succeed as a hairdresser, it's important to be genuinely enthusiastic about the job. Hairdressing requires commitment and plenty of stamina, but with a positive attitude you'll find that the rewards far outweigh any downfalls. (Chapter 6 will tell you more about the qualities you need to be a good hairdresser.)

Quick recap!

- ✓ The developments in the hairdressing industry in the 1960s had a profound effect on hairdressing today.
- ✓ The Hairdressers (Registration) Act 1964 gave hairdressers official recognition as a body of professionals.
- ✓ Most hairdressers hold a relevant hairdressing qualification.
- ✓ According to the City & Guilds Happiness Index, hairdressers are the happiest workers of all.

CHAPTER 3
REAL LIVES 1

ZAK RANSON: JUNIOR STYLIST

Zak Ranson is a junior stylist at Toni & Guy in Muswell Hill, north London. He has worked in the salon for two years and is about to complete his NVQ2 qualification. In a few months' time, he will spend six weeks at the Toni & Guy Academy in central London to gain their diploma and become a stylist.

'I've been interested in hairdressing ever since I can remember. I enjoyed messing around with family members' hair when I was a kid, and I liked creative subjects like drawing at school. But the real inspiration for me was my cousin. She has her own hairdressing business and is an ambassador for Toni & Guy products, introducing them to other salons.

'She advised me to apply for a job here after I left school. She knew Toni & Guy offer really good training and that they're well respected in the industry. So I applied for a junior's job in this salon – it was advertised in the shop window. They asked me to send in my CV and attend an interview, and I had to do a trial day in the salon so they could assess whether I'd be right for the job. I was really pleased when they decided I would be.'

Zak had already done some work experience in a hairdressing salon when he was at school. He'd gone to college once a week to study for NVQ entry level, which involved a mixture of theory and practical work and included a two-week block in a salon. There he'd learned basic skills like blow drying and washing hair. Those skills helped prepare him for his role as a junior.

'I wash clients' hair, make them drinks and supply them with magazines, tidy the salon and ensure a steady stream of clean towels. It means I'm on my feet all the time except for when I have a break – we get an hour for lunch and have a 15-minute break in the morning and the afternoon.

'Now that I'm more experienced I also help with the blow drying. And because I've been here longer than the other juniors, I show new assistants around the salon and check that they're doing what they should be. They know they can come to me if they've got any questions.

'Normally we work from 9.45am to 6.30pm, although we finish at 8pm on Thursdays. On Saturdays we work from 8.15am to 5.30pm. It tends to be quieter at the beginning of the week but Wednesdays, Thursdays and Fridays are usually busy and Saturdays are hectic! It can be tiring but you get used to it.'

Zak has been studying NVQs since he joined Toni & Guy. Along with the other juniors, he stays late in the salon on Monday and Wednesday evenings to be trained by the qualified staff, who teach on a rotating basis. They cover cutting techniques on Mondays and colour techniques on Wednesdays, which means they need a constant supply of models to practise on! They also need to cover the theory. To ensure they're maintaining the right standards, an NVQ assessor comes in once a month to assess their performance.

'I was quite nervous the first time I cut a model's hair, but I quickly built up confidence and it comes easily now. It was the same with colour. Once I've attended the Toni & Guy Academy next year I'll be qualified to cut hair on the shop floor. You specialise in either cutting or colour for your diploma and my specialism will be cutting hair. I think it's a very creative skill and I'm excited about doing it.

'I love working and learning in a salon; nothing beats the hands-on experience. You're dealing with proper clients and standing next to stylists, observing what they do and listening to what they say. A really important part of this job is advising clients on what suits them. We cover that in our NVQ course but we learn a lot about it from the stylists too. We also learn time management skills. Clients are booked in for specific time slots and it's important to keep to those as much as you can.'

> 66 You've got to be able to talk to people and take an interest in clients, and that comes naturally to me now. 99

Zak says a big plus of the job is its sociability – you meet clients from every walk of life and can build up close relationships with your colleagues.

'We all get on well with each other here. When it's someone's birthday we'll go out for a meal, and we keep in touch with people after they leave. I was a bit shy when I first came here, but this job really brings you out of your shell. You've got to be able to talk to people and take an interest in clients, and that comes naturally to me now.

> **66** I think [hairdressing] is a very creative skill and I'm excited about doing it. **99**

'Because I came here straight from school, I wasn't prepared for the intense training and the long hours. I also had to get used to working on Saturdays, although that doesn't stop me going out in the evening with my mates! It's well known that the pay isn't brilliant when you start, but there's the potential to earn considerably more when you start working as a stylist.

'For me it's all about doing something that I really love. Hairdressing can take you anywhere and you can do so much with it – I'd eventually like to go out to salons and teach cutting techniques. I'd also like to own my own business, like my cousin.

'To anyone considering a career in hairdressing, I'd say "go for it" if it's something you really want to do. Remember, appearance is everything – hairdressers make clients look better and so they need to be presentable themselves.'

> **Zak's top tip**
> **66** When you go for your interview, dress smartly, take an interest and ask lots of questions. **99**

CHAPTER 4
WHAT ARE THE JOBS?

Provided you're prepared to work hard and take the time to learn the trade, you'll find hairdressing offers plenty of opportunities.

Most hairdressers work in salons, which can range from small, independently owned businesses to large chains such as Toni & Guy. In a small salon, the hairdressers do most of the work themselves, including sweeping up hair and making tea for clients. In larger salons which employ more staff, an assistant will normally carry out these tasks for the hairdressers.

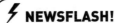 **NEWSFLASH!**

Hairdressing is traditionally a hierarchical industry, which means you have to be prepared to start at the bottom and work your way up.

You might be itching to get your hands on those scissors, but no reputable salon would allow you on the floor with clients until you'd proved your ability to do the job. And while you need the right training to be able to progress (see Chapter 10 for more), seasoned hairdressers all agree that qualifications are no substitute for practical experience.

The good news is that once you've put in the groundwork and gained that all-important experience as a stylist – preferably at a senior level – hairdressing can open up an exciting array of options, many of which weren't available 20 or 30 years ago.

As well as the option of going freelance and choosing the hours you work – which can be invaluable if you've got a young family – modern hairdressing extends into everything from styling models' hair for the catwalk to working on a cruise liner and travelling the world.

> **"** . . . modern hairdressing extends into everything from styling models' hair for the catwalk to working on a cruise liner and travelling the world. **"**

Once you've entered the profession, you'll find the career route roughly follows the stages outlined below, although job titles are likely to vary. (You'll find information about salaries in Chapter 8.)

SALON OR BARBER ASSISTANT

This is the role in which nearly all hairdressers 'cut their teeth' in the profession. The basic duties might include sweeping up hair, greeting clients and answering the phone, making tea, washing hair and handing things like rollers to stylists.

Assistants can normally expect on-the-job training; many combine the job with study for NVQ/SVQ 1 and 2, perhaps under an Apprenticeship scheme or as part of a salon's training programme (see Chapter 10). This enables you to practise styling and cutting techniques on mannequins and models before moving on to 'real' clients.

LEARN THE LINGO
Don't know what a word means? Turn to the Jargon Busters chapter on page 101 to find out.

As an assistant, you may be asked to wash clients' hair. This will help you to recognise different types of hair and to work out which shampoos and conditioners are best suited to them. Product knowledge is an important part of the job, as every modern salon uses (and often sells) a variety of products, from conditioning treatments to mousses. To perform your job effectively, you'll need to know what each one does and the best way of using it. You may also be asked to blow dry clients' hair; again, you'll learn to do this in a professional way. Part of an assistant's role is to learn from the stylists, and this is one of many areas where you can benefit from observing them at work.

Another key part of the job is learning and demonstrating basic health and safety procedures, from disinfecting combs to cleaning mirrors and shelves after the salon closes. These are some of the first things you'll learn when you start work in a salon, and they will also be an essential part of your formal training.

JUNIOR STYLIST, BARBER OR AFRICAN-CARIBBEAN HAIRDRESSER

This is the next rung up the ladder. As a junior, you'll be able to move on to the salon floor to perform basic cutting, styling, setting, colouring and drying techniques. That means you'll be carrying out consultations with clients and advising them on which products will best suit their hair.

You'll probably also be mixing and applying strong chemicals for basic colouring and perming, so you'll need to put your knowledge of health and safety into practice. This will include carrying out skin tests to determine whether a client has an allergic reaction to products like hair dyes. It will also mean keeping a careful track of time so you don't ruin a client's hair by leaving strong products in it for too long. In addition, you may need to diagnose hair and scalp conditions (head lice are not uncommon).

> 66 As a junior, you'll be able to move on to the salon floor to perform basic cutting, styling, setting and drying techniques. 99

Most salons are unisex, which means you'll be dealing with male and female clients. If you've chosen to work in barbering, now is the time you'll need to perform additional services such as shaving and trimming beards. And if you're in a salon that specialises in Afro-Caribbean hairdressing, you'll need to start carrying out specialist techniques like plaiting, braiding and relaxing hair.

Unless you're in a very small salon, you'll be working as part of a team and your duties will probably overlap with those you carried out as an assistant. You may, for example, be asked to cover reception duties and work on the till. As a junior you can usually expect some supervision. These days, it is usual for salons to require juniors to have an NVQ/SVQ level 2 qualification in hairdressing or barbering.

SENIOR STYLIST, BARBER OR AFRICAN-CARIBBEAN HAIRDRESSER

To become a senior hairdresser or barber, you'll need to have had plenty of experience on the salon floor. You'll normally have to demonstrate skill in all aspects of modern hairdressing, including advanced techniques for cutting, styling and colouring. You'll be expected to build your own clientele and may be required to perform specialised services like dressing and accessorising hair for special occasions.

Many senior staff train and supervise juniors, although you'll normally need an NVQ/SVQ3 for this. (Some larger salons help their staff work towards this qualification.) Senior hairdressers or barbers may also help managers and

> ⚡ **NEWSFLASH!**
> A single human hair has an average lifespan of between three to seven years.

salon owners recruit new people. In larger salons, they may become involved in such things as fashion shows and salon publicity activities.

This isn't to say they won't also have more mundane tasks to perform. If a senior stylist works in a small salon, they'll probably still need to 'muck in' with tasks like ordering stock, operating the till and cashing up earnings. And even if it's a larger salon, they may need to perform duties like mixing chemicals and putting in foils for highlights and lowlights.

> ❝ If a senior stylist works in a small salon, they'll probably still need to 'muck in'. ❞

Once you reach this level of expertise, however, you'll be able to consider other options, such as going freelance.

SALON MANAGER OR OWNER

Once they've become fully fledged hairdressers – which is likely to take several years – many people go on to start up their own salon. This can be highly satisfying, and many salon owners 'keep their hand in' by continuing to work on the floor with clients.

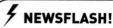

NEWSFLASH!

Whatever your position in the hierarchy, you'll need to stay alert to jobs that need doing and play your part in helping the salon run smoothly.

However, running a salon is a competitive business and, as you'll read in Chapter 6, the demands of being a salon owner or manager are quite different from those of being a stylist. You'll need to undertake a range of additional responsibilities, from stock control to marketing the salon, and you'll have to understand and apply such skills as business planning and financial management.

Selling retail products like waxes, mousse and conditioning treatments could well be an important source of income, so you'll need to ensure that your staff have a good knowledge of the products on offer and that they're able to recommend them to clients. (There's currently a need for retail selling skills within the industry.) In addition, running a salon involves recruiting and managing staff: if someone is off sick, for example, it's down to you to find the best way of keeping the salon running smoothly.

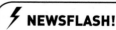

NEWSFLASH!

Hairdressing is dominated by small, privately owned businesses, many of which are managed by their owners.

Some people opt to manage someone else's salon, although in both cases it's preferable to have specialist training (see Chapter 10). It's also worth noting that opportunities to manage a salon are more limited than opportunities to work as a stylist.

GOING FREELANCE

A popular option for an accomplished hairdresser is to go freelance: over 40% of hairdressers and barbers are self-employed. Some work from home, with clients coming to visit them there. Others become mobile hairdressers, travelling out to clients' homes or to places like hospitals and care homes to work with patients and residents.

TOP TIP!

If you're a mobile hairdresser, it's essential to have a valid driving licence.

As a freelance, you could also rent a chair in a large salon and book in your own clients. And, as in hairdressing generally, the key to success is establishing and maintaining a warm relationship with clients – providing a good service so they'll keep coming back for more.

If you go freelance, you'll need to make your own appointments, build your own client base, and order your own stock and equipment. As a self-employed person, you'll be taxed differently from an employee, so you'll also need to keep an accurate record of your earnings and outgoings.

OTHER HAIRDRESSING JOBS

The range of jobs available to hairdressers and barbers has mushroomed in recent years. Some workplaces employ hairdressers directly, on either a permanent or a sessional basis; others lease out premises to salons or barber shops. You could be based in a department store, a hospital or care home, a holiday resort or even an airport.

Your careers adviser will be able to tell you more about the different jobs available, but they include the following.

Cruise liner hairdresser or barber

This is a popular option and recruitment standards are high – you'll need to be fully qualified and it's preferable to have salon experience (check recruitment requirements with individual companies). There can be high demand for blow drying and hair styling skills because of the formal evenings on board. Most cruise liners offer a good social life and benefits like free meals – and, of course, free travel! It's usual to be paid on a commission-only basis – again, check the details with individual companies.

> 66 Most cruise liners offer a good social life and benefits like free meals – and, of course, free travel! 99

Film or TV hairdresser

This involves styling hair for people who will appear on camera, either on location or on a film set in a studio. Hairdressers work closely with colleagues in the make-up and costume departments, and the work can include dressing and applying wigs and hairpieces as well as creating both modern and period styles. Despite the often long hours, this type of work is much in demand. Applicants need NVQ/SVQs up to level 3 and should be willing to travel and live away from home.

Session hairdresser

Being a session hairdresser is another highly sought after area of work. It involves styling models' hair for photo shoots, whether for commercial TV adverts, magazines or the catwalk. This could take you anywhere from a photographer's studio to a deserted rural village, and you'd be working closely with design teams and photographers to achieve a co-ordinated look. Although this type of job sounds glamorous, the hours can be long and the work intense. Salaries are substantial, especially for commercial film work.

HM prison hairdresser or barber

You could be cutting or styling hair for prisoners or wardens, or you could train prisoners in hairdressing or barbering skills. This work can be highly fulfilling but isn't for the inexperienced. You'd need to pass a security check into your background before you could start the job.

Armed forces hairdresser or barber

You could work in a salon or barber's shop on a military base, providing a service for people for live or work there. Again, you'd be required to undergo a security check.

Platform artist

A platform artist demonstrates hairdressing techniques to an audience, often from within the hairdressing trade. You could find yourself in front of anything from 100 to 2000 people. As you'd expect, this isn't a job for beginners: it demands full qualifications, experience, excellent communication skills and steady nerves! However, you can earn good money and the job can take you to both national and international locations.

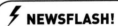 **NEWSFLASH!**

Salon tipping is always at the customer's discretion, but 10% to 15% is considered the norm if you think you've received good service.

Teaching, lecturing and assessing

Many hairdressers enjoy sharing their skills with others, either in a salon environment or in a college. To teach in a salon you'll normally need NVQ level 3, and college lecturers will need a Further Education Teacher's Certificate as well. This usually takes up to two years to complete. Some hairdressers combine part-time teaching with running a salon.

Hairdressers with at least two years' experience and NVQ3 can also take QCF Assessor/Assessment Qualifications. This equips you to observe, assess and guide people working towards NVQs in a variety of workplaces, including salons. You can also develop relationships with employers, youth organisations and schools.

RELATED FIELDS

Hairdressing also offers the potential to move into related fields, including:

▶ working in **research and development**

▶ **selling and promoting** hairdressing products for manufacturers

▶ providing **technical advice** in areas like colouring and perming

▶ **trichology**: helping people with hair and scalp disorders

▶ making **wigs** for theatre companies.

It's worth noting the increasing overlap between the hair and beauty therapy industries. Hairdressers working in television and theatre, for example, also need make-up experience, and spas and holiday resorts may require hairdressers to carry out procedures such as manicures.

⚡ **NEWSFLASH!**

A human hair is stronger than copper wire of the same thickness.

Salons are also increasingly diversifying into everything from electrolysis to spa treatments. To competently carry out beauty therapy treatments, you need specialist training, and this is widely available. The new Diploma in Hair and Beauty Studies (see Chapter 10) covers both hairdressing and beauty therapy and is an excellent launching pad to specialised study in either area.

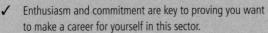

Quick recap!

✓ You must prove your ability to do the job before you are allowed to cut clients' hair.

✓ Enthusiasm and commitment are key to proving you want to make a career for yourself in this sector.

✓ As an assistant, you'll be expected to learn from a stylist, so ask lots of questions and be aware of what is going on around you.

✓ Remember, there are lots of great opportunities available once you have the relevant qualifications and hairdressing experience. You can work overseas, teach, or even work in the army!

CHAPTER 5
REAL LIVES 2

LINDA LANDER: FREELANCE HAIRDRESSER

Linda Lander works from her south London home as a freelance hairdresser. She became a hairdresser relatively late in life, at the age of 40, and worked for over seven years in a salon. She has been self-employed for just over 10 years.

'I always wanted to be a hairdresser but became a PA after I left school. In those days people thought you only went into hairdressing if you couldn't do anything else.

'It was only years later, when I was having my hair cut in a local salon, that someone mentioned it ran evening classes. I thought: "It's now or never" and went and enrolled.'

It was the best move Linda could have made. She studied the salon's in-house diploma for two evenings a week plus Saturdays over 18 months. It was a big commitment but it meant she was still able to work during the day. She then started working part time in a salon and completed her NVQ2 and NVQ3, also on a part-time basis.

'I discovered I had a flair for hairdressing, and working in the salon meant I could do something I loved but still find time for my children. I also taught in the salon's school.

NVQs were widely available by that time and I trained part-timers towards NVQ2, for which the salon was an accredited centre.

'Although I really enjoyed the work, I decided to go freelance because it gave me more flexibility. But it was quite tough at first: being self-employed isn't as easy as people think. You have to be well-organised – the skills I'd learned as a PA came in useful – and you have to be self-motivated and disciplined. That means getting up in the morning and telling yourself, "This is a work day" even if you feel like sitting out in the garden!

> 66 The really good thing about this type of work is that you can fit it around your other commitments. 99

'It took me about three years to really get established. Ordering stock was a learning process to begin with: I got better at it when I worked out which products I got through more quickly. I buy direct from the suppliers now.

'The really good thing about this type of work is that you can fit it around your other commitments, although you do have to be flexible to suit other people. On an average day I might see five clients, but it can vary – I might see seven on one day and two on another. Some I see every five weeks, others I might see once a year.

'I've never advertised and get all my clients through word of mouth. I give out my phone number, but never my address, as I'm working from home and cut hair for men as well as women.

'I've set up a room in my house as a mini-salon and do all my work from here. That's never been a problem, as a lot of women want to go out to have their hair done. It's also suited me: I could be there for my daughter, who was still quite young when I started, and I have everything to hand. The downside is that people can expect you to be on tap 24 hours a day.

'I put my qualifications up on the wall so that clients can see that I've got them. They can also see I'm state registered, which I think should be mandatory in this country. Hairdressers work with strong chemicals and it's important to know what you're doing.

'When I was in the salon, I learned advanced cutting and colouring techniques and that's stood me in good stead. My specialism is colouring hair, although I still do a lot of cutting. I also use some of the barbering techniques I learned, such as razoring. On my NVQ course we learned razoring by shaving a balloon and it was great fun.

'It takes hard work to make a success of going freelance, but I'd do the same again. Although I make a good living from it, it's a way of life as much as a job. One of the best parts for me is meeting people from so many walks of life. You have to be a good listener, but it's great when you can make someone's day better. You also have to keep up to date with trends and colours: I have a lot of young clients, and I need to know what they're talking about when they ask for a particular style.

'Hairdressing opens the door to other things as well. I've done a couple of hair shows, including one for my NVQ3, when I demonstrated how you can adapt 1950s hairstyles for the present day. I've styled wigs for pantomimes and amateur dramatic events, and last year I went to Germany to do the hairstyles for a wedding party.

'I definitely wouldn't advise anyone to go out on their own until they've got salon experience: you'd miss out a whole chunk of the learning process. One of the first things you learn is how to do a consultation, and it's invaluable to see how salon stylists do it. You can also watch how they approach different things and bounce ideas off each other. If a client's made a mess of dyeing their hair, what's the best way of putting it right? I still have friends in the trade who I ask for advice.

'To anyone who wants to be hairdresser, I'd say stick at it and the world can be your oyster. Approach it as if you were going to college or university: you won't earn much to begin with, but if you work hard and think outside the box, it can give you a good living and a lot of satisfaction.'

Linda's top tip

❝ A hairdresser needs to be confident, but not too confident: It's important to recognise when you might need a second opinion. ❞

CHAPTER 6
TOOLS OF THE TRADE

Scissors, combs and brushes are just some of the tools we expect hairdressers to use – and becoming skilled in using them is clearly an essential part of the job.

But anyone who's made it in hairdressing will tell you it takes a lot more than technical skill to get on in this profession. In hairdressing, you have to start at the bottom and work your way up, and that takes dedication and a lot of hard work.

Providing a streamlined service to clients can seem deceptively easy, but it takes a huge amount of practice. You have to make them feel at ease, conduct a consultation and provide a professional cut or treatment – all within an allocated time slot. That's why no reputable salon would let you work as a stylist until you'd served your time as an assistant and proved your ability to do the job.

While solid training will give you the right foundations (see Chapter 10 for more), you'll be much better equipped to make a go of hairdressing if you possess certain personal qualities. It's worth adding, too, that the qualities you need to become a good stylist won't necessarily equip you to run your own salon or employ other people.

LEARN THE LINGO
Don't know what a word means? Turn to the Jargon Busters chapter on page 101 to find out.

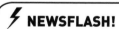

Take a look at the personal tools of the trade outlined in the next few pages to work out whether you have them or could develop them, perhaps through work experience or a Saturday job in a salon.

COMMUNICATION SKILLS

Hairdressing is all about people – it's a service industry that revolves around making clients look and feel good. So if you want to get on in this industry, you'll need to be able to communicate with people of a wide variety of ages and backgrounds.

If you've been to a salon yourself, you know what it's like to be a client: you expect the hairdresser to ask you questions, put you at ease and deliver a good result. Even the quieter ones will do their best to ensure you're happy with their work. If that hasn't been your experience, how likely would you be to go back or to reward the hairdresser with even a modest tip?

⚡ NEWSFLASH!
A fascinator is a popular hair accessory. It consists of decorations like feathers and flowers attached to a comb, clip or headband. Women usually wear it at the side or front of the head.

That's why the ability to establish a rapport with clients is essential in this business – and being able to chat about anything from the weather to the price of eggs is a definite plus.

But don't worry if you're not naturally 'gabby'. One of the most important attributes of a good hairdresser is to be a good listener. You'll also need the ability to interpret a customer's requests. If someone with shoulder-length hair comes in and asks to have it cut short, do they mean to the bottom of their neck or to behind their ears?

While the ability to make small talk can increase with practice and confidence, you need a genuine interest in people to succeed in hairdressing. If the thought of hearing about a client's trip to Benidorm or how their boyfriend fell asleep in the bath fills you with horror, you need to think seriously about whether hairdressing is really for you.

> **66** One of the most important attributes of a good hairdresser is to be a good listener. **99**

TACT

Another essential skill is the ability to be tactful. When people go to a hairdresser, they want to feel good as part of the experience. So if you tell them that having a cropped cut will make their ears stick out even more, they may not return in a hurry!

Part of being tactful is to listen encouragingly to what clients want and to suggest workable alternatives if you think they're being unrealistic. Clients often ask hairdressers for their opinion and attach a lot of importance to what they say. That means it's up to you to respect that trust and be sensitive to their feelings. While being honest is important, that rarely means telling the whole unvarnished truth. It's also important to learn to recognise when clients don't want you to volunteer an opinion.

Again, your ability to read people and deal with them tactfully will

> ⚡ **NEWSFLASH!**
> The beehive hairstyle, associated in our times with singer Amy Winehouse, takes its name from the tall structure of a beehive. It was hugely popular in the 1960s.

increase with experience. The important thing is having the interest and patience to keep working at it.

DEXTERITY

As a hairdresser, you need the ability to work quickly and accurately with your hands. This is a practical job that requires skill in using everything from scissors to waxes and hairdryers. Although you can learn the technical skills of the trade, it will help a lot if you have manual dexterity to begin with.

AN EYE FOR DETAIL

Having a keen eye for detail is also important. Ensuring, for instance, that you've cut a client's hair evenly on both sides of their face is a key part of doing the job properly. Again, you can develop this skill but if you're naturally slapdash you might be better suited to a job that requires less precision.

STAMINA

As a hairdresser, you'll be on your feet a lot of the time and will probably have to work long hours. During peak times, a typical salon is a busy environment: you'll be talking to people continuously, often without a break, and will need the ability to multi-task. That means you'll need stamina and a good level of physical fitness to cope with the demands of the job.

> **66** As a hairdresser, you'll be on your feet a lot of the time and will probably have to work long hours. **99**

TEAM WORKING

In most salons hairdressers work as part of a team, with a hierarchy of people from assistants to stylists to managers, so you'll need to work closely together to provide a good service. If you're the salon assistant, for example, you'll need to help stylists by providing drinks for the clients and sweeping up hair.

BEING POSITIVE AND ENTHUSIASTIC

Giving a good impression to clients is paramount in this profession, so it's important to appear positive even if you're having a bad hair day yourself. While this may involve some degree of acting, it shouldn't mean putting on an Oscar-winning performance every time someone walks through the door. To last the course as a hairdresser, you'll need to have genuine enthusiasm for what you're doing. You'll also need to be willing to learn new methods and techniques, as this industry is constantly changing to keep up with customer demand.

You need to do everything to the best of your ability, from shampooing a customer's hair to answering the phone. It's all part of your development – and if you're a good cleaner, the chances are you'll be a good hairdresser!

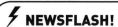 **NEWSFLASH!**

Sweeney Todd, the fabled 19th-century barber of Fleet Street, was reputed to cut his clients' throats with a razor, rob them and turn them into meat pies.

CREATIVITY

You don't need to be a born artist to become a good hairdresser, but it helps to have creativity and an artistic

> 66 To last the course as a hairdresser, you'll need to have genuine enthusiasm for what you're doing. 99

sense. When you're cutting or colouring someone's hair, you'll be paying attention to form and to how the colour blends in with their overall appearance. While you'll normally cover these things on a training course, you'll have a head start if you have natural flair.

APPEARANCE AND PERSONAL HYGIENE

This industry is all about making clients look good, so it's important for the people providing the service to be well-groomed and presentable themselves. It's also important to have good personal hygiene. Remember you'll be in close contact with clients – touching their hair, leaning across them and looking into their faces.

TOP TIP!

Bad breath and dirty fingernails are definitely out!

KEEPING CALM

As we've said already, a typical salon can be a hectic environment, with pressure to keep within allocated time slots and to meet clients' expectations. There can also be added pressures such as clients complaining or arriving late, or even electricity cuts.

Not only that, but many clients see the salon as a sanctuary from the pressures of their everyday lives. They're looking for a relaxing and rejuvenating experience, which is why it's common for assistants to massage a client's head when they're applying conditioner. It's therefore important for you to be able to manage your own stress levels and to convey a sense of calm to your client. While you'll become better at this with practice, if you find it hard to keep calm under pressure this may not be the right job for you.

> 66 As a manager, you'd need to be extremely well-organised, with good team-building and problem-solving skills. 99

TIME MANAGEMENT SKILLS

Doing a good job within an allocated time slot is what hairdressing is all about, and you'll get better at this with practice. But time management also extends to punctuality – arriving on time and not keeping customers waiting (if this is unavoidable, you'll need to ensure someone offers them a drink or a magazine). If you're a night owl, you might have to cut back on your social activities to ensure you're in good form for the next day's work.

LEARN THE LINGO
Don't know what a word means? Turn to the Jargon Busters chapter on page 101 to find out.

GOING THE EXTRA MILE

Many hairdressers dream of eventually running their own salon, and a lot go on to do it. However, as we said earlier, running a salon requires additional skills you might not possess as an assistant or stylist. Foremost among these will be such skills as business planning and salon marketing and, if you're employing other people, you'll need a thorough knowledge of employment law and recruitment practices.

Many colleges and universities run courses, some at degree level, to equip people with expertise in these areas. However, running your own business is extremely demanding and takes a high degree of motivation, dedication and self-discipline. To make a real go of it, you need to be willing to put 100% into it.

Managerial skills

Before taking the plunge, you might find it helpful to manage someone else's salon, which would give you valuable experience and help you decide whether you really want to branch out on your own. As a manager, you'd need to be extremely well-organised, with good team-building and problem-solving skills. You'd also need the commitment to undertake a range of other responsibilities, from stock control to maintaining a client database, which would require good IT skills. (Although around 50% of salons still use paper-based records, computer use is rising.)

As you saw in the previous chapter, however, many hairdressers opt to become self-employed without being business owners. Their work can range from travelling to people's homes to renting a chair in a salon and booking in their own clients. Although you'll need much the same qualities as any hairdresser for this type of work, you'll be making your own bookings, buying your own stock and equipment and handling your own finances – so you'll need good planning and numeracy skills.

It's worth bearing in mind, too, that this type of work is more solitary than being employed in a salon, so you'll need the ability to work on your own initiative. That also applies to more glamorous-sounding jobs like working on fashion shoots and TV commercials, which demand drive and stamina, as well as plenty of experience.

OTHER THINGS TO CONSIDER

Attention to health and safety is one of the first things you learn as a hairdresser – and it's for your protection as well as other people's. You'll be working with powerful chemicals, from bleaching agents to perming lotions, and if you're prone to skin irritations or breathing problems it might be wise to seek advice from your doctor before starting a career in hairdressing.

Also, as discussed earlier, you'll be on your feet for most of the day and this might not be a good idea if you've got back problems. The demands of working in a salon don't combine easily with raising young children either, although many women, in particular, return to hairdressing when their children are older or continue with it on a part-time basis.

> ## ⚡ NEWSFLASH!
>
> The American hippy musical *Hair* opened in London on 27 September 1968, one day after theatre censorship was abolished. Until then, some of its scenes – which included drug taking and nudity – would not have been allowed on a stage in Britain.
> *Source: news.bbc.co.uk/ onthisday*

Now you know the sort of person you need to be to succeed in hairdressing, read on to discover how other people are doing it.

Quick recap!

✓ In hairdressing you have to start at the bottom and work your way up.

✓ You need to be able to establish a good rapport with your clients to be a successful hairdresser.

✓ Salons operate well if the staff work well as a team.

✓ Remember, clients expect you to be well-groomed and professional.

CHAPTER 7
A DAY IN THE LIFE
OF A HAIRDRESSER

SACHIYO KOYAMA: SALON OWNER

Sachiyo Koyama is joint proprietor of Alfie's in Stukeley Street, central London. She and her business partner, Harry, both work in the salon full time and employ one other hairdresser, who is also full time. Sachiyo worked in London salons for eight years before setting up her own business. She previously trained as a hairdresser in Japan, where it's mandatory to be fully qualified before working with clients. She worked in salons there for 18 years before coming to England.

'We're open for six days a week, from Monday to Saturday. Our normal opening time is 10am, although we're prepared to be flexible to suit customers. If we're doing clients' hair for a wedding party, for instance, we might open an hour earlier. We'd charge a bit extra for that.

'I usually come in at about 9.30am to set everything up, although we'll often swap around so that one of us can come in a bit later. One of the first things we do is to switch on the boiler for hot water. It's also important to ensure that the window facing the street is clean. Because we don't employ an assistant or receptionist, we need to do all the paperwork and cleaning ourselves. On a typical day I'll be cleaning up every 10 minutes: sweeping the floors, checking the trays and doing whatever else needs to be done.

'It's usually quieter at the beginning of the week, although it gets busier towards the end, and Fridays and Saturdays are our peak times. It also tends to be quieter in the mornings. If I'm not with a client, I'll often sit at reception, taking phone calls and doing the books. I'm constantly checking our stock to see what we need to re-order. It could be anything from foils for highlights to shampoo or conditioner. I order in new colour supplies every two weeks, usually 25 to 30 different tints each time. All our hair products come from Wella and Redken; I used them when I was employed as a hairdresser and I'm familiar with how they work.

'On a typical day I might see five clients, although I could see nine on a busy day. More people come in for a cut than anything else, especially men, although we offer the full range of treatments, including colour. Most of our clients are regular – some followed us here when we set up our business – but we also get a lot who walk in from the street. This is a cosmopolitan area and I love the fact that we have an international clientele. Some clients come in every week, others every few months. A lot work in the area or are students nearby; we also have a few older women who come in for a shampoo and set.

'A cut and blow dry normally takes about an hour, although I'll allow up to two and a half hours for highlights or a major colouring job. That's including a consultation, which could take five minutes if the client is asking something straightforward but longer if they want a major style change or if I need to work out what to do. I'll do the consultation before the client puts on their gown. That helps me to assess how their hairstyle will fit in with their overall appearance. It also helps to know what type of job they do. Someone who works in an office, for instance, might want a different look from an actress.

'Clients will often ask what colour suits them best, and that's where my experience comes in; it takes a lot of practice and technical knowledge to get it right. But what I'm most in demand for is my cutting technique. The other day, a woman came in who'd seen a lady on a bus with a haircut she liked. She was looking for a new hairdresser so asked where she'd had her hair cut, and the lady had recommended me! I gave her a cut and she seemed pleased, so I hope she'll become a regular client.

'Building a good customer base is one of the most rewarding parts of the job for me. I know immediately whether a client is happy with my work from the look on their face. If they're happy, I'm happy: providing client satisfaction is what this job is about. There are a lot of hairdressers in the world and it's great when a client chooses you.

'What I find most difficult is when clients aren't clear about what they want, or if they come in with unrealistic expectations. They might bring in a picture from a gossip magazine and want to look exactly like a celebrity, and I need to be tactful in suggesting that another style might suit them better. Technique, instinct and taste are the three things I've really developed in this job.

'We don't close the salon until 7 to 7.30pm, sometimes later, and we have to clear up and lock up before we leave. It's a long day and it's very hard work, but I love it. I wouldn't have the same degree of satisfaction if I was still working for someone else. And one of the good things about it is that you don't take your work home with you on a BlackBerry. Once you go home, your work is finished for the day.'

CHAPTER 8
FAQs

By now you'll be getting a feel for hairdressing – the size and range of the profession, the types of job available and the qualities you'll need to 'cut it' as a hairdresser. Hairdressing is all about making people look and feel good, but what can you expect to get out of it as a career? What are the prospects and what will it mean for you personally? This chapter answers some of the most commonly asked questions about hairdressing and should help you decide whether this really could be the career for you.

 Q 🙶 **How much will I get paid?** 🙷

A There are no set rates of pay, but once you're qualified as a stylist you can expect to earn £13,995 per year upwards – and you'll be able to command more as you gain experience. A lot will depend on where you work. Wages in big cities, especially London, are higher than in less urban areas.

It's no secret, however, that you won't earn a great deal when you start out. Many trainee hairdressers earn around the national minimum

> ## ⚡ NEWSFLASH!
>
> The annual British Hairdressing Awards, established in 1985, have significantly raised the profile of British hairdressing both in the UK and abroad. Previous winners of the prestigious British Hairdresser of the Year award include Trevor Sorbie, Anthony Mascolo, Charles Worthington and Beverly C.
>
> *Source: www.britishhairdressing* 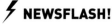 *awards.co.uk.*

wage, which will vary according to age and hours worked but is likely to range from around £7,000 to almost £12,000 per year. If you're doing an Apprenticeship, you'll receive a minimum of £95 a week, although many employers pay more than this. Many hairdressers find it easier to make ends meet if they live at home during this early period, when it's important to take time to learn the trade.

LEARN THE LINGO
Don't know what a word means? Turn to the Jargon Busters chapter on page 101 to find out.

The good news is that as you progress through the profession, the amount you earn can increase dramatically. An experienced senior stylist might end up earning over £30,000 per year, and if you go on to manage a salon, work as a platform artist or style hair for catwalk shows you can expect to earn considerably more than that (although you'll need to put in the hours).

If you go freelance you'll be setting your own rates, but the Freelance Hair and Beauty Federation recommends a minimum of £25 per hour.

And those who go on to lecture in a college could expect to earn from £26,000 to £32,000 per year in London, although the salary will vary according to length of service and location.

Don't forget, too, that it's established practice for clients to tip hairdressers if they're satisfied with the service, and if you're a good hairdresser those tips can make a difference (although you will be expected to pay tax on them). Some salons pay commission on top of your basic salary; a good stylist could earn 30% to 40% of their service takings. Some salons also pay commission on retail products that you sell.

Q **What hours will I work?** 99

A Most hairdressers work around 40 hours a week, but this isn't spread evenly throughout the week. Saturday is the busiest day and you'll almost certainly need to work then, although you'll probably have a day off during the week to make up for it. Most salons open late on one or two evenings a week (often Thursday and Friday), although they may close early at the beginning of the week.

You'll need to bear in mind that your service will probably be most in demand at times you might want to be out with your friends, such as Friday evenings. Although a few larger salons may operate a rota system, smaller salons (and these are by far the majority) will usually need all hands on deck, especially in busy times such as the run-up to Christmas, when a lot of clients will want their hair styled.

66 To find out whether hairdressing really could be for you, it's a good idea to get a Saturday job or a work experience placement in a salon. 99

There's also an increasing trend for salons to extend their opening times to coincide with clients' out-of-work hours, and it's common for staff to work overtime to cover these periods. Most salons don't open much before 9am on a weekday, which is good news if you're not an early bird – but do expect an earlier start on Saturday to accommodate the numbers of clients coming in.

Many salons take on part-time staff, which is an important point to bear in mind if you're thinking of starting a family. Many also employ extra staff on a Saturday.

 Q 66 **How much time will I get off for holidays?** 99

A This will vary according to the salon – but employers normally allow 28 days a year, including public holidays (this has been a legal requirement since April 2008). Bear in mind, however, that there will be less flexibility to take time off during busy periods, especially Christmas and the New Year, and some salons may expect you to take at least some of your holiday at predicted quieter times, such as February. If you're self-employed, you can arrange both your holidays and hours to suit yourself, although you'll probably want to make yourself available during times of high demand.

66 What qualifications will I need? 99

For some years, the standard recognised qualification in the industry has been the National Vocational Qualification (NVQ), or Scottish Vocational Qualification (SVQ) in Scotland. However, this isn't the only qualification you can take, there is also the Diploma in Hair and Beauty Studies. (You can read more about qualifications in Chapter 10.) At present, you normally need to be qualified to at least NVQ level 2 before you can work as a stylist, and level 3 is the industry standard. Some salons help their staff to gain NVQs, for example through the Apprenticeship scheme.

Once you're qualified to at least NVQ level 2, you can register with the Hairdressing Council on a voluntary basis, which gives you recognition within the industry.

  66 How do I get started? 99

To find out whether hairdressing really could be for you, it's a good idea to get a Saturday job or a work experience placement in a salon. It will give you practical experience, which is crucial in this industry, and will help to build up your confidence and people skills. As we've said already, hairdressing, like barbering, is very much a people profession, and being able to talk to clients and work as part of a team are essential elements of the job.

NEWSFLASH!

Hairdressing takes its name from the centuries-old art of dressing the hair – styling or arranging it to achieve a particular effect.

Remember, too, that hairdressing is an industry where appearances count, so make sure you're well turned out and that you arrive at the salon on time. Employers will want you to be willing to learn and to have plenty of enthusiasm, so demonstrate these qualities in everything you do – from sweeping up hair to making tea for customers.

If you're interested in getting an Apprenticeship, ask your careers adviser or local Connexions service whether they know of local salons which are looking for recruits. You can also register with the National Apprenticeship Service on www. apprenticeships.org.uk (see Chapter 10 for more).

Before you begin a specific qualification in hairdressing (see Chapter 10), it can be useful to have GCSEs. However, commitment and eagerness to learn are equally, if not more, important.

TOP TIP!

Once you've learned the ropes and qualified as a stylist, it's likely to take you at least a couple more years to move into a senior stylist's role.

Q
A

66 What are the prospects? 99

As you'll have read in Chapter 4, hairdressing is quite a hierarchical industry, which means you have to be prepared to start at the bottom and work your way up. But if you're willing to learn and to work hard, there are plenty of progression opportunities – from running a salon to going freelance and choosing the hours you work.

Hairdressing these days is a highly professional industry and it takes time and plenty of practice to become really accomplished at it. But once you've gained experience and proved you have the ability and perseverance to succeed, you can expect a progressive salon to offer you further opportunities. Not only that, but hairdressers with highly developed technical skills are in demand, so you're unlikely to be out of a job.

Joining a trade association can help to keep you in touch with developments. If you're ambitious, it's worth bearing in mind that there are plenty of competitions you can enter, many sponsored by major product names. You'll find a lot advertised in trade magazines (see Chapter 13).

TOP TIP!

This isn't a profession that stands still, so to stay at the 'cutting edge' you'll need to retain an active interest in the industry – staying alert to new trends, attending refresher courses, networking at trade fairs and exhibitions.

There are currently technical skills shortages in areas like long hairdressing, colour correction and African-Caribbean hairdressing, while in barbering there's a demand for skills like shaving, face and scalp massage and hair relaxing techniques. There are also shortages in salon management and business planning skills, and in associated areas like recruitment, marketing and selling retail products. This means that if you can carve a niche for yourself in these areas your skills are likely to be in high demand. There's also a continuing demand across the board for good stylists.

> 66 You can transfer the skills you gain in hairdressing to other industries or take them with you around the world. 99

For highly skilled and experienced hairdressers, the sky really is the limit. There are opportunities to move from the salon floor into areas like teaching, being a platform artist, working on TV and fashion shoots, and creating hairstyles for catwalk shows. These jobs can potentially earn you good money, although they frequently involve long hours and aren't as glamorous as they're cracked up to be.

You can transfer the skills you gain in hairdressing to other industries or take them with you around the world.

Q 66 **What will I get out of it personally?** 99

A Many professional hairdressers say there's nothing like the buzz you get from helping someone look and feel better. A skilled and creative hairdresser can actually make a difference to people's lives, which is a highly rewarding experience. It's also very satisfying to be in demand for a quality service that people feel is worth paying for.

Q 66 **Where will I work?** 99

A The most likely place is a salon, whether this is in a big city, a small town or a largely rural area. There's a demand for hairdressers everywhere and most people don't want to travel too far to reach one. That means you'll find salons and barbers' shops in most places where people live and work.

CAREER PROGRESSION OPPORTUNITIES

ASSISTANT
SALON ASSISTANT OR BARBER ASSISTANT

↓

JUNIOR
JUNIOR STYLIST, BARBER OR AFRICAN-CARIBBEAN HAIRDRESSER

↓

SENIOR
SENIOR STYLIST, BARBER OR AFRICAN-CARIBBEAN HAIRDRESSER FREELANCE HAIRDRESSER OR BARBER CRUISE LINER HAIRDRESSER OR BARBER FILM OR TV HAIRDRESSER HM PRISON HAIRDRESSER OR BARBER ARMED FORCES HAIRDRESSER OR BARBER RELATED WORK SUCH AS INDUSTRY SALES AND MARKETING

↓

EXPERT
SALON OWNER OR MANAGER SESSION HAIRDRESSER PLATFORM ARTIST LECTURER

However, as you'll have read in Chapter 4, hairdressing offers the opportunity to work in a range of other places, from care homes to department stores. As you gain experience, a broadening range of job options is likely to open up to you, and these could take you anywhere from travelling the world on a cruise liner to working on location in the Bahamas (or a muddy field in Essex!) for a film shoot.

Q 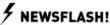 **Will I be able to work abroad?** 🙶🙶

A Yes, there's a wealth of opportunities for UK-based hairdressers to work abroad, from plying your trade in holiday resorts to working in international hotels. There's also the opportunity to travel the world with a cruise liner or long-haul airline, although competition for these jobs is fierce.

⚡ **NEWSFLASH!**

Rinsing the hair in sage tea and apple cider vinegar is reputed to stimulate growth.

Within Europe, it's a case of 'have qualifications, can travel'. NVQs and SVQs in hairdressing are recognised right across the European Union, so if you have these qualifications to at least level 3 standard you should be able to work in EU countries without the need for further training.

Beyond Europe, Habia – the UK government-approved body that sets standards for the industry – has developed Habia International Qualifications (HIQs) for the international market. Like NVQs and SVQs, HIQs are directly related to the competencies employers require in the workplace and are recognised in a number of countries. Habia is working to achieve worldwide recognition for its standards so that anyone with a qualification based on these standards will be able to practise hairdressing abroad without the need for further training.

 Check it out!

Find out more from the Habia website (www.habia.org/international).

It's worth adding that the UK hair industry enjoys a good reputation internationally for its standards and creativity. A number of other UK hairdressing qualifications, including City & Guilds and BTEC qualifications, are widely recognised in other countries, as is the government-backed State Registration Certificate, which is available to all qualified hairdressers. You can find out more about that from the Hairdressing Council website – www.haircouncil.org.uk.

If you choose to take up the opportunity to work abroad, there's no doubt that it will expand your horizons and expose you to different cultures. English is widely spoken across the world and you may not need another language, especially if you're working for a British company. However, a working knowledge of other languages will never be wasted. Being able to speak even a little of your host country's language will help to signal an interest in their way of life and is likely to go down well with local clients.

Q

A

66 **Will working with chemicals be a problem?** 99

It may well be if you have sensitive skin, allergies or asthma. As a hairdresser you'll be exposed to strong chemicals, mixing them together to apply to clients' hair and breathing in the fumes. Even if you don't suffer from skin allergies, it's important to follow health and safety guidelines – and these are some of the first things you'll learn in a salon.

The Health and Safety Executive (HSE) estimates that up to 70% of hairdressers suffer from some form of work-related skin damage during the course of their career; this is nearly always preventable. (See www.hse.gov.uk/hairdressing for more.)

Habia also campaigns to raise awareness about dermatitis and to promote the use of gloves. Take a look at their comprehensive health and safety section on www.habia.org.

⚡ **NEWSFLASH!**

The classic short 'bob' became popular in the 1920s. At first cut straight all round the face, often with a fringe, it has been reinvented ever since, notably by Vidal Sassoon in the 1960s. Celebrities like Victoria Beckham and Keira Knightley have brought it back into the spotlight with a modern twist.

Q **How easy is it to join a salon and train in-house?**

A Not all that easy, although positions do exist. There's stiff competition for in-house training schemes in large salon chains like Vidal Sassoon and Toni & Guy, especially as these groups represent only around 2% of hairdressing outlets. However, a number of smaller chains and larger salons also offer in-house training schemes. A great many of these, including the ever-popular Apprenticeships, enable you to complete NVQs and SVQs while you're working.

TOP TIP!

If you're applying for an in-house scheme, always find out whether it's recognised within the industry.

It's also a good idea to increase your chances of being offered a place by gaining work experience in a salon first, perhaps through work experience or a Saturday job. To get on an in-house scheme, you'll have to attend an interview and may be asked to spend a few hours in the salon to demonstrate your willingness and ability to perform basic tasks.

Q **Where can I find out about vacancies?**

A When you're ready to apply for a job, you'll find vacancies advertised in local and national newspapers, on hairdressers' websites, and in Job Centre Plus offices. You can also find out about job opportunities through your Connexions centre and local salons.

Quick recap!

✓ You won't be earning a very high wage when you enter the hairdressing industry but once you start to progress, your salary can increase dramatically.

✓ You might not be able to take time off when other people traditionally take their holidays, such as Christmas and New Year, as these are likely to be a hairdresser's busiest periods.

✓ Because of the specific technical skills held by hairdressers, you are unlikely to find yourself out of work.

✓ Remember, tips from clients can make a big difference to your salary so it's really important to always provide a fantastic service.

CHAPTER 9
REAL LIVES 3

SOPHIA HILTON: STYLIST

At the age of 21, Sophia Hilton has already worked in a series of salons and won 17 hairdressing medals. She'd started her A levels, one in fashion, when she realised she was more interested in hair than clothes. So she left school after taking her AS levels and did NVQ2 and 3 at college, working in salons during her spare time.

'My mum and nan owned a salon in Blackpool, which was initially a deterrent. I used to sweep up and shampoo hair and thought it was boring.

'But I took to hairdressing easily when I realised it was what I wanted to do; I've always been artistic and it's actually very creative. My college tutor entered students into junior hairdressing competitions, and I won a gold and bronze medal in the Lancashire Championships for bridal hair. They were the first competitions I'd entered and it made me think: "I could be good at this." '

Sophia left college but kept entering competitions, averaging one every two months for two years. She worked in a salon as a junior stylist for three days a week to ensure she kept learning, went freelance for one day and reserved the fifth day for competition entries.

'Because I came from a small town, it made me want to do big things. One of the competitions I won was the World Skills regional competition for juniors (up to age 25). I went on to gain second place in the national competition and was put into the British team for the international World Skills competition.

'It's the largest international vocational skills competition in the world – it's run by the government and features every trade in the country. The judges pick a winner from every trade and they represent Britain in the international championships, which are held in a different country every year. I was teamed up with people from a whole range of areas – from landscape gardening to hospitality services. I'm still good friends with a florist I met. I trained intensively with coaches for seven months, which was a great experience. Although I didn't win a place on the international team, it got me where I wanted to be.

> **❝** Whenever a new job comes up in the salon, even if it's something uninteresting, I'll show initiative and put myself forward. **❞**

'I applied for a job in Manchester in the chain salon Regis and got it; I was 19 and they made me style director. That wouldn't have happened without my World Skills experience or my practical salon experience.'

Six months later, when she was helping out with the hairstyling at a wedding exhibition in her spare time, Sophia met a student photographer and started working with him on photo shoots. They invented about nine shoots and had some published in *Hairdressers Journal International* and *The Hairdresser*, produced by the Hairdressing Council. They also moved to London together.

'I took the first job that came up, which was in a good salon. But I wanted the opportunity to get involved in other things, such as fashion shows and event co-ordination. Although I love hairdressing, I don't want to stay on the floor for longer than five years. That's why I chose Brooks & Brooks salon in Holborn, whose work encompasses everything from seminars to filming for DVDs.

'I was very persistent – I sent in my CV twice and left my portfolio with them for a week. But the turning point was when the owner recognised me from a competition I'd entered. I hadn't won it but she was sufficiently impressed to invite me to an interview. They offered me a job as a graduate stylist; it's not a grand sounding title but their standards are very high and my boss is inspirational.

'Whenever a new job comes up in the salon, even if it's something uninteresting, I'll show initiative and put myself forward. That's why I get asked to do more interesting things – it's about give and take. I've just been helping out with demonstration work, travelling round to wholesale suppliers to show them new products. You do the demos in front of an audience of about 30 people.

'It's important to stop your hands shaking when you do seminar or show work, which is why my boss is giving me this experience now. Although I'm a confident person, it takes practice; you can get very nervous when the whole room is watching. My boss has been a platform artist for 20 years and still gets nervous.

'There's really so much you can do with hairdressing, but you do have to be prepared to slog it for a while at first. You also need plenty of floor experience before you can

> 66 There's really so much you can do with hairdressing, but you do have to be prepared to slog it for a while at first. 99

go on to things like floor shows. If you're ambitious, make it your aim to be the best at every stage – the best shampooer, the best blow dryer, the best stylist.

'Even if you're not ambitious you can make a great career out of it. You do need good physical endurance; we used to laugh when they told us to stand with our legs apart in health and safety lessons, but it was for a reason. You're on your feet all day with your hands raised, and your back can hurt if you're not careful. People aren't always prepared for that when they move into hairdressing full time after doing it as a Saturday job.

'I'd like to see more academic kids go in for hairdressing. Although it's come a long way, it can still be seen as a bit of a dropout career. But I had other options and chose hairdressing, and it was the best thing I could have done.'

CHAPTER 10
TRAINING AND QUALIFICATIONS

The world of hairdressing today is very different from 20 years ago – and nowhere is this more apparent than in the field of training. Today, there is such a wealth of qualifications available in hairdressing that it can be confusing to work out what they are and how they relate to one another. A big plus of the system, however, is its flexibility – wherever you are in the UK, you can usually find a qualification that meets your needs. The information below is intended as a general guide. Your careers adviser will help you look at what's available locally and find a qualification that's right for you.

Habia, the government-appointed standards-setting body for qualifications in the hair and beauty sector, points out that hairdressing qualifications can be divided into two broad types: job ready and preparation for work.

JOB-READY QUALIFICATIONS

Job-ready qualifications, as the name suggests, equip learners to show they are able to work to the relevant National Occupational Standards for their job; and that they are therefore competent in their occupation. National Vocational Qualifications (NVQs), which are the recognised industry qualifications in hairdressing (see below), are an example of job-ready qualifications.

PREPARATION-FOR-WORK QUALIFICATIONS

Preparation-for-work qualifications, on the other hand, are broad qualifications based around vocational and transferable skills. They do not give competency, but do provide you with a sound practical and academic foundation – preparing you for the further training and experience you'll need to become job ready. The new Diploma in Hair and Beauty Studies, which is now available in many schools and colleges in England (again, see below), is an example of a preparation-for-work qualification.

LEARN THE LINGO
Don't know what a word means? Turn to the Jargon Busters chapter on page 101 to find out.

While employers have traditionally expressed a preference for job-ready qualifications, ideally Apprenticeships, the Diploma aims to develop wider skills for an ever-expanding workforce, providing the general skills you need to succeed at work as well as depth and breadth of subject knowledge. Many employers believe that this will lead to more well-rounded individuals entering the workplace.

You can study for hairdressing qualifications in a variety of ways: through a full-time or part-time school or college course, perhaps with work release; as part of an Apprenticeship; or on day or evening release as part of a salon's own training scheme.

You can contact your local college or training provider to find out about available courses; your careers adviser will be able to help. You can also find out more from Connexions (www.connexions-direct.com), the Department for Education (www. education.gov.uk) and Habia (www. habia.org). Before you embark on a course, especially if you're paying for it at a private college, check with your careers adviser or Habia that it's recognised within the industry.

> 66 One of the most popular routes into hairdressing is through an Apprenticeship, which enables you to work in a salon and study for a level 2 or 3 NVQ/SVQ at the same time. 99

While you don't need specific qualifications to get into hairdressing, it helps to have GCSE passes, especially in maths or English. The new Diploma in Hair and Beauty Studies will enable you to decide whether this is really the sector for you before you undertake an industry-specific NVQ or SVQ course. Again, your careers adviser will be able to point you in the right direction.

To make it easier to compare one qualification with another, all have been assigned to an educational level. The Qualifications and Credit Framework assigns the level at which each one is recognised in England, Northern Ireland and Wales. Level 1, which is equivalent to GCSE grades D to G, is the most basic, although you can also take an entry-level certificate to prepare you for learning at this level. Industry figures show that while over 60% of hairdressers have a level 2 qualification – which is considerably higher than the national average – they are far

Check it out!
You can search for accredited hairdressing qualifications on www.accreditedqualifications. org.uk.

less likely to be qualified at level 4 or above. Employers hope that clearer progression routes from level 1 to level 4 and beyond will help to change this pattern.

NVQs/SVQs

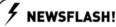

⚡ NEWSFLASH!

The average scalp has over 100,000 hairs.

For many years, the recognised industry standard for hairdressing has been the National Vocational Qualification (NVQ) or Scottish Vocational Qualification (SVQ). NVQs/SVQs are practical, work-based qualifications which are broken down into a series of units that enable you to learn and build upon each of the skills you need to become a competent hairdresser or barber. They are measured through on-the-job assessment, so if you're studying them at school or college you'll need access to a work placement.

There are three main levels of NVQs/SVQs (but there are five levels overall).

1. **Level 1** is an introduction to the industry, with a level of competence geared to a salon trainee, and is available only in hairdressing.

2. **Level 2** equates to a junior stylist and enables you to use chemicals and work unsupervised. It is available in hairdressing and barbering.

3. **Level 3**, which equates to senior stylist level, covers advanced techniques and enables you to handle the books and train other staff. Again, it is available in both hairdressing and barbering.

The widely accepted minimum qualification for hairdressing is NVQ/SVQ level 2, and it normally takes up to two years to reach this level. However, employers are increasingly expecting staff to be qualified to level 3, which is now the industry standard. There are no age restrictions or minimum entry requirements to study for NVQs/SVQs, although for level 1 some colleges may give preference to applicants with one or two GCSEs (A* to C) or Key Skill passes.

However, personal qualities are considered more important than qualifications. Some young people aged 16 or over progress to NVQ level 1 from an Entry to Employment (E2E) scheme, which prepares you for employment by helping you learn job-related skills such as team working. Your careers adviser will be able to point you in the right direction.

APPRENTICESHIPS

One of the most popular routes into hairdressing is through an Apprenticeship, which enables you to work in a salon and study for a level 2 or 3 NVQ/SVQ at the same time. Crucially, you earn as you learn – the minimum entitlement is £95 a week, although some salons pay considerably more.

To be eligible for an Apprenticeship, you have to be aged between 16 and 24 years old and not in full-time education when you apply. Apprenticeships are available in England, Northern Ireland, Scotland and Wales, although they have different titles in all four nations.

▶ In England you can take an Apprenticeship and Advanced Apprenticeship.
▶ In Northern Ireland you can take level 2 ApprenticeshipNI and level 3 ApprenticeshipNI.

- ▶ In Wales you can take a Foundation Modern Apprenticeship and Modern Apprenticeship.
- ▶ In Scotland you can take a Modern Apprenticeship.

They are available in either hairdressing or barbering. Although there are slight differences in the frameworks for each of the four nations, all Apprenticeships incorporate both a work-based qualification (NVQ/SVQ) and transferable or 'key/core/essential/functional' qualifications, including maths, English and ICT, which you take with a local training provider.

There are three levels of apprenticeship available.

1. **Intermediate:** at this level you would work towards a level 2 NVQ or a BTEC.
2. **Advanced:** at this level you would work towards a level 3 NVQ or BTEC.
3. **Higher:** at this level you would work towards either a level 4 NVQ or a Foundation degree.

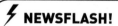 **NEWSFLASH!**

Hair is the fastest growing tissue in the human body next to bone marrow.

As an apprentice, you'd spend most of your time in the workplace alongside experienced staff. You'd also be assigned a mentor through your local training provider, who would liaise with your employer and develop a learning plan for you. You'd typically be working for 36 to 42 weeks in a year.

You can apply for and start an Apprenticeship at any time of the year, but be warned – competition is fierce! Some salons will advertise Apprenticeships and you can apply to them direct. You can also contact the National Apprenticeship Service, which has a vacancy-matching service, or speak to the work-based learning co-ordinator at your local college or training provider, who may have a list of employers who are looking to take on an apprentice.

Although there are no specific entry requirements, you'll need to attend an interview and undertake an initial assessment: employers will be looking for commitment and enthusiasm. Some young people progress to an Apprenticeship from an Entry to Employment (E2E) course. Again, your careers adviser will be able to point you in the right direction. You can normally complete an Apprenticeship in between 18 months and three years depending on your previous experience.

> 66 There are currently skill shortages in areas like salon management, so if you're looking to spread your wings into management, these could be for you. 99

YOUNG APPRENTICESHIP

If you're aged 14 to 16 years old, have good motivation and expect to attain at least five GCSEs at A* to C level, a Young Apprenticeship in Hairdressing might be for you.

Young Apprenticeships combine classroom learning with on-the-job learning. As well as continuing to study the school curriculum, you'll have the opportunity to spend 50 days over a two-year period working in a salon, which will give you a good flavour of what hairdressing is like. You'll also work towards a level 2 vocational qualification (not an NVQ) for two days a week. One of the beauties of a Young Apprenticeship is that it enables you to keep your options open: you can still decide to opt for A levels or a different area of work. You'd also be well-equipped to move on to an Apprenticeship (see above).

Your teacher or careers adviser will know whether your school offers Young Apprenticeships. If it doesn't, you may be able to do the vocational qualification part of the Young Apprenticeship at a local college.

DIPLOMA IN HAIR AND BEAUTY STUDIES

The Diploma, which is a government initiative, represents one of the biggest reorganisations of education for 14- to 19-year-olds in England in the past 50 years. (Diplomas are not yet available in all parts of the UK.) Since September 2009, the Diploma in Hair and Beauty Studies has been available in a number of areas in England through consortia of schools, colleges and training providers. It is set to be a national entitlement by September 2013.

> ⚡ **NEWSFLASH!**
>
> A traditional hair remedy to add shine to dark hair is to use diluted vinegar in the final rinse.

The Diploma is available in three stages: Foundation, Higher and Advanced.

- ▶ The Foundation Diploma is equivalent to five GCSEs at grades D to G.
- ▶ The Higher Diploma is equivalent to seven GCSEs at grades A* to C.
- ▶ The Advanced Diploma, which includes management and business skills for the hair and beauty sector, is equivalent to three and a half A levels.

In 2011, a Progression level will also be available. This will be the equivalent to two and a half A levels and is for those who do not wish to continue with an entire Advanced Diploma.

Because the Diploma in Hair and Beauty Studies covers all six industries within the sector – hairdressing, barbering, African-type hair, nail services, spa therapy and beauty therapy – it provides a broad overview which should give you a head start in your future career.

The Diploma also equips you with a range of skills and knowledge that enable you to make an informed choice about what to do next. Once you've completed the Foundation or Higher Diploma, you can go on to:

▶ study the Advanced Diploma

▶ study other types of qualification such as GCSEs, A levels or NVQs (you can also study GCSEs and A levels while you're doing the Diploma)

▶ do an Apprenticeship

▶ move into employment with training.

An important element of the Diploma is applied learning. This brings together academic and vocational learning by allowing you to develop specialist knowledge, skills and understanding about the industry through practical workplace tasks. These are all relevant to real work in the hair and beauty sector.

You will have the opportunity to investigate areas of particular interest, such as hair colouring, through the specialist learning options. You can also opt to include GCSEs or A levels. In addition, all Diploma students are required to cover the skills they will need for successful future learning and employment. These include personal learning and thinking skills and functional skills in maths, English and ICT.

A major objective is to develop 10 key skills which employers want new recruits to have. These are:

1. communication
2. creativity
3. customer care
4. flexible working
5. leadership

6. personal and professional ethics
7. positive attitude
8. self-management
9. team work
10. willingness to learn.

⚡ NEWSFLASH!

British women have their hair done more often, and spend on average 20% more doing so, than women anywhere else in the world.

Source: www.guardian.co.uk/ lifeandstyle/2008/jan/09/ fashion.shopping.

Because it is geared to giving learners the understanding, skills and mindset they will need to succeed in both work and further learning, the diploma has received widespread support from the hair and beauty sector.

If your school does not currently offer the Diploma in Hair and Beauty Studies, it is likely that another provider in your area will be able to help. Ask your careers adviser for advice or visit the Diploma website on www.diplomainhairandbeautystudies.org.

To find out more about vocational programmes outside England refer to the awarding bodies listed in Chapter 13.

VOCATIONALLY RELATED QUALIFICATIONS

You can also take a number of Vocationally Related Qualifications (VRQs) in hairdressing. VRQs are like NVQs in that they are designed to develop your employment skills. Unlike NVQs, however, they provide a broad introduction to an area of work, focusing on what you know and understand rather than on what you can do. As such, they can be a good preparation for NVQs, Apprenticeships or employment.

Two VRQs used as part of the Young Apprenticeship scheme, for instance, are the Certificate in Hairdressing (level 2) offered by the Vocational Training Charitable Trust (VTCT) and the City & Guilds level 2 Diploma in Women's Hairdressing Services. Other widely recognised VRQs are the BTEC National Certificate and National Award in Hairdressing (both level 3), which give you a good grounding in the knowledge and skills needed in the hairdressing industry. Both these qualifications foster problem-solving and applied learning skills, helping you develop an understanding of the industry through practical workplace tasks. Learners often progress to one of these awards from an NVQ2 or a BTEC National Certificate.

Your careers adviser will be able to tell you more about VRQs and how they dovetail with other industry recognised qualifications.

LEVEL 4 AND ABOVE

Once you've gained plenty of experience in the industry, you might want to work towards more advanced qualifications. There are currently skill shortages in areas such as salon management, so if

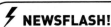

NEWSFLASH!

Fewer than a quarter of women who are born blonde keep this hair colour naturally after their teenage years.

you're looking to spread your wings into management, these could be for you. Both NVQ/SVQ level 4 and City & Guilds Higher Professional Certificate or Diploma in Technical Salon Management (also level 4), for example, are specifically geared to salon management.

In England, a number of higher education institutions offer Foundation degrees (levels 4 to 5) in salon management and related areas such as human resource management. Like NVQs, Foundation degrees have been designed by the industry for the industry to ensure that they're relevant to the workplace.

To be considered for a Foundation degree, you normally need an A level, a BTEC National Certificate in Hairdressing or an NVQ level 3 in Hairdressing, but entry requirements vary so check with individual providers. UCAS will have a list of institutions that offer Foundation degrees; see Chapter 13 for contact details. Foundation degrees usually take a minimum of two years to complete.

CONTINUING DEVELOPMENT

Although Britain is one of the few nations where you don't need recognised qualifications to practise as a hairdresser, once you've got NVQ/SVQ level 2 you can apply to become a State Registered Hairdresser through the Hairdressing Council (see Chapter 13). Becoming a State Registered Hairdresser will give you professional standing within the industry, as well as recognition as a hairdresser under UK law.

> **TOP TIP!** *i*
>
> You can keep up to date with what's going on in the profession by attending short courses – City & Guilds run short awards in areas such as colour correction and hair extensions.

In addition, hairdressing is an industry where you never stop learning, as new products and techniques are continuously coming onto the market.

You can attend trade fairs and demonstrations in different parts of the UK. Self-employed hairdressers can benefit from the short courses offered by the Freelance Hair and Beauty Federation (FHBF); these range from

ACCESS TO HAIRDRESSING

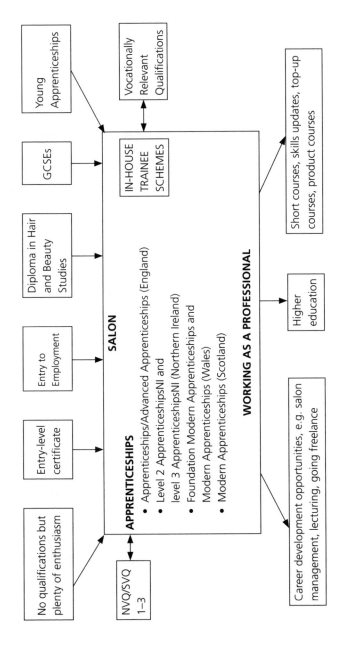

running a mobile business to bridal hair. You can also keep at the cutting edge of developments in the profession by subscribing to a trade journal. See Chapter 13 for contact details.

NATIONAL OCCUPATIONAL STANDARDS

Habia has developed a set of National Occupational Standards (NOS) for the hair and beauty sector in association with employers, educators, industry professionals and trade bodies.

These standards underpin the range of accredited qualifications in the sector for levels 1 to 3, including NVQs/SVQs and Apprenticeships. They describe what people need to do, know and understand to carry out their jobs to a competent standard and can help learners identify training needs and career routes.

There are separate standards for hairdressing, barbering and African-type hair as well as for beauty therapy, nail services and spa therapy.

You can find the full range of standards on the Habia website – www. habia.org

Quick recap!

✓ Apprenticeships are generally considered to be the best way to enter the hairdressing industry.

✓ While there are no set qualifications to get into hairdressing, it's useful to have GCSEs in maths and English.

✓ The new Diploma in Hair and Beauty Studies is widely supported by hairdressing professionals.

✓ Remember, personal qualities and dedication to learning on the job are every bit as important as qualifications.

CHAPTER 11
REAL LIVES 4

DAVID BARRON: SALON OWNER AND MANAGER

David Barron owns and runs Barrons on Muswell Hill Broadway, North London. He employs a team of 10 to 12 people: a reception/salon-co-ordinator, stylists and trainee assistants. David has built his reputation as an innovator, combining hairdressing and photography skills. As well as winning the Innovation of the Year award at the 2000 British Hairdressing Business Awards, he has won a string of hairdressing and photography awards and his photographs have been published nationally and internationally.

'My father died suddenly when I was 13 years old and from then on I knew I'd have to make my own way in life. School for me was like trying to run through treacle and I couldn't wait to leave. Consequently, I left school at 15 years old without any qualifications, and as hairdressing was in my family I decided to learn the trade. Little was I to know that I'd embarked on what was to be my education and a world of opportunity. That was in 1965 and my first job was as an assistant at a barber's shop in Soho, London. It was a bit Dickensian and for about 10 shillings a week I was expected to work six days a week from 8am to 8pm.

'I moved on to Benny Raymond's barber's shop in Marble Arch. There I was introduced to precision cutting by Benny's son Victor and learned the exacting skills and techniques of men's hair cutting, from short back and sides to American crew cuts – all done with no electric tools, just scissors, combs and cut-throat razors and within a 20-minute maximum slot. It was at that time that I recognised the potential of men's hairdressing.

> 66 A lot of today's hairstyles reflect a retro 60s look – everything eventually turns full circle. 99

'Towards the end of the 1960s, the young fashion-conscious men wanted longer hair and hairstyles had become more unisex. I started developing different styles and techniques to keep men's hair longer. A lot of today's hairstyles reflect a retro 60s look – everything eventually turns full circle.'

When David was 19 years old, he applied to Steiner's to work as a barber on a cruise liner. He relished the opportunity of travelling the world and was offered a job on *RMS Franconia*, which took passengers on cruises to the Mediterranean, America and the Caribbean.

'I remember turning up at Southampton in December 1968 and being overwhelmed by the size of a 30,000 ton ship. I was given a barber's shop with two chairs all to myself to run. Next door was the ladies' salon, and when they saw how I cut hair, they asked me to cut their hair. They also asked me to train them to cut women's hair.

'But the really big breakthrough for me was discovering I could communicate with people from all walks of life. I changed overnight from a confidence-lacking teenager to someone who realised the world was their oyster. While I was on the ship I also became inspired by photography. I'd become good friends with the ship's photographer and realised that he got the first look in with the pretty young girls as they came on board: he took their pictures as they were greeted by the ship's captain.'

David returned to London to work in a Steiner's salon near Victoria station, where he continued to style hair for both men and women.

'At that time London was swinging; I remember the Rolling Stones giving a concert in Hyde Park, with Mick Jagger wearing a white dress. Then one of my cousins, who worked in a barber's shop in Barnet, north London, asked if I wanted to go there during my leave to earn some extra money. He said I wouldn't know what had hit me when I started work in the suburbs, and he was right: I did a week's holiday relief hairdressing and it was incredibly busy. They asked me to show them how I cut hair, and that inspired me to start my own business.'

> 66 The *Hairdressers Journal* used to come down almost every week to see what we were doing and take pictures, which were featured regularly in both the men's and ladies' pages. 99

David saw a small hairdressing shop in Hornsey, north London, advertised for sale in the *Hairdressers Journal*. The asking price was £300 – the amount he'd been able to save while working on the ship. (His wage had been £9 a week, but his board and lodging had been free.) The shop needed a facelift and the seller accepted his offer of £275, which enabled him to buy some paint and get some cards printed.

'I called the salon One Step Ahead, painted the inside and outside black with the help of my friends and put up photos which were a bit risqué. I thought they were artistic, but shortly afterwards the local papers reported that some local residents had complained and they put a picture of the salon on the front page.

'As a result, we were overflowing with people who flocked to the salon. It was new and innovative, we were trendy and played rock music, we did funky haircuts for men and, soon after, for women as well. The *Hairdressers Journal* used to come down almost every week to see what we were doing and take pictures, which were featured regularly in both the men's and ladies' pages.'

> 66 Good cutting is the bedrock of modern hairdressing as it's developed over the past 40 years, and the course emphasises precision cutting. 99

Five years later, David moved One Step Ahead to Muswell Hill and opened a hairdressing school in his Hornsey premises. Three years after that, in 1977, he moved to new premises on Muswell Hill Broadway and opened Barrons Hairdressing & Photovision, which offers customised photography as well as hairdressing.

'I've re-introduced my own training course into my salon, and would like to get it accredited so I can take it further afield. Good cutting is the bedrock of modern hairdressing as it's developed over the past 40 years, and the course emphasises precision cutting. There's also an emphasis on practical aesthetics – height, head and face shape, the way the hair grows, hair type – and communicating with people as individuals, which is an essential skill for any hairdresser.

'Hairdressing has become glamorised in today's world, but it's still a profession where you have to learn on the job. A lot of young people come into the salon with the illusion that they're ready to be a stylist just because they've been to a hairdressing college and got an NVQ2 qualification in hairdressing.

'I'm all in favour of having recognised qualifications – I think they should be compulsory for hairdressers in this country – but hairdressing has to be learned from experience. As a salon owner I wouldn't let anyone loose on my clients unless they'd proved that they could meet my standards.'

David's top tip

❝ To be a successful hairdresser, you have to be willing to learn; however long you've been doing the job, you never stop learning new skills. As hairdressers, we work in a privileged industry. It's important for anyone in hairdressing to realise that we have an opportunity to make a difference to how people feel about themselves; the experience of coming to a salon should be uplifting and inspiring. It goes without saying that a hairdresser or technician must have the technical ability to achieve the best hair results for each client. But it's equally important that they're able to communicate verbally in a genuine and professional way in order to go 'beyond hairdressing'. **❞**

CHAPTER 12
THE LAST WORD

If you've read through this book, you'll have seen the variety and fascination that a career in hairdressing can offer. This is a dynamic and high-profile industry that's progressed in leaps and bounds over the past 20 years. There are now excellent training and development opportunities, with the chance to branch out into other areas once you've proved that you've got what it takes.

Hairdressing is an industry that never stands still: there's a constant stream of new techniques and products coming onto the market, from funky colouring treatments to state-of-the-art styling aids. But one thing that definitely won't go out of fashion is the demand for good hairdressers. Even during the recession, salons have vacancies to fill, and as the economy recovers the industry is sure to become even more buoyant.

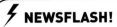

⚡ NEWSFLASH!
Smokers are four times more likely to have grey hair than non-smokers.

As the case studies in this book have shown, hairdressing can offer huge personal satisfaction. It isn't for nothing that City & Guilds Happiness Index surveys have found hairdressers to be the UK's happiest group of workers. If you've reached the conclusion that this might be the career you're looking for, you'll find the following chapter a useful source of information. It contains contact details for key bodies in the sector, including professional and training organisations. But first take a minute to answer the questions in the checklist below. They should help you decide if you're on the right track.

THE LAST WORD

Tick yes or no

Do you enjoy talking to people?	☐ Yes	☐ No
Are you a good listener?	☐ Yes	☐ No
Are you enthusiastic and positive?	☐ Yes	☐ No
Are you excited about learning new things?	☐ Yes	☐ No
Do you enjoy working with your hands?	☐ Yes	☐ No
Do you enjoy working with people?	☐ Yes	☐ No
Have you got plenty of stamina?	☐ Yes	☐ No
Do you take pride in your own appearance?	☐ Yes	☐ No

If you answered 'YES' to all these questions, then congratulations! You've chosen the right career. If you've answered 'NO' to any of these questions then this may not be the career for you. However, there are plenty of other jobs within hairdressing that might suit you better, such as being a receptionist in a salon, selling hair products or marketing.

CHAPTER 13
FURTHER INFORMATION

In this chapter you'll find contact details for relevant industry, training and government bodies. They are presented in alphabetical order. A good place to start is Habia – www.habia.org (see below).

ORGANISATIONS

City & Guilds
1 Giltspur Street, London EC1A 9DD
Tel: 020 7294 2800
www.cityandguilds.com

City & Guilds is the UK's largest awarding body for vocational qualifications. It offers a range of hairdressing qualifications including Apprenticeships, NVQs and SVQs, Key Skills, Higher Level Qualifications and City & Guilds vocational qualifications.

City & Guilds has joined forces with AQA, the UK's main provider of GCSEs and A levels, to offer a range of diplomas, including the Diploma in Hair and Beauty Studies, which require a combination of academic and vocational learning. You can find out more from the AQA–City & Guilds Diploma website – www.diplomainfo.org.uk.

Connexions

www.connexions-direct.com

The Connexions website is aimed mainly at 13- to 19-year-olds but contains a wealth of job-related information that could be useful to a range of age groups. Click on Jobs4U for the careers database and then the A–Z Search to find specific information about being a hairdresser.

Directgov

www.direct.gov.uk

Directgov brings together in one place information and online services on every aspect of public life. The employment section includes details about the national minimum wage (NMW) and the Education and Learning section includes information about Diplomas. You'll find job profiles for a range of careers, including hairdressing, on www.careersadvice.direct.gov.uk.

Edexcel

190 High Holborn, London WC1V 7BH
Tel: 0870 240 9800
www.edexcel.com

Edexcel is the leading provider of internationally recognised qualifications. It is the sole provider of BTEC qualifications including BTEC Certificates, Nationals and specialist and short course qualifications in hairdressing. It is also one of the providers of the Diploma in Hair and Beauty Studies.

Freelance Hair and Beauty Federation (FHBF)
The Business Centre, Kimpton Road, Luton LU2 0LB
Tel: 01582 431783
www.fhbf.org.uk

The Freelance Hair and Beauty Federation is a non-
profit-making organisation that represents the interests
of freelance hairdressers and beauty therapists in the
industry. It offers its members benefits, services and training
opportunities.

Habia
Oxford House, Sixth Avenue, Sky Business Park, Robin Hood
Airport, Doncaster DN9 3GG
Tel: 0845 230 6080
www.habia.org

Habia is the government-appointed standards-setting body
for the hair and beauty sector. It creates the standards that
form the basis of all qualifications in the sector as well as
industry codes of practice. The Habia website contains a
wealth of information on everything from careers to
health and safety. You can find specific information about
diplomas on www.diplomainhairandbeautystudies.org.

Hairdressing Council
30 Sydenham Road, Croydon CR0 2EF
Tel: 020 8760 7010.
www.haircouncil.org.uk

The Hairdressing Council maintains an official register
of qualified hairdressers and campaigns for registration
to become a legal requirement. It also runs hairdressing
competitions and advises consumers.

Health and Safety Executive (HSE)
Tel: 0845 345 0055
www.hse.gov.uk

The HSE is a government body that works to protect people from health and safety hazards in the workplace. You'll find information and advice about preventing dermatitis on www.hse.gov.uk/hairdressing.

Learning and Skills Council
Apprenticeship helpline: 0800 015 0600
www.lsc.gov.uk

The LSC is a non-departmental government body set up to improve the skills of young people and adults. It plans and funds all post-16 education in England outside the universities. For Apprenticeships, go to the A–Z list on the homepage or visit www.apprenticeships. org.uk. Apprenticeships in hairdressing are listed under Types of Apprenticeships – Retail and Commercial Enterprise.

For Modern Apprenticeships in Scotland, visit www.careers-scotland.org.uk or www.modernapprenticeships.com.

For Apprenticeships in Northern Ireland, visit www.delni. gov.uk/apprenticeshipsni

National Database of Accredited Qualifications
www.accreditedqualifications.org.uk

You can search this site for accredited courses in England, Wales and Northern Ireland.

National Hairdressers' Federation (NFH)

One Abbey Court, Fraser Road, Priory Business Park,
Bedford MK44 3WH
Tel: 0845 345 6500
www.nhf.info

Membership is open to all salon owners and self-employed
hairdressers who work in a salon. The NFH supports and
represents its members in a variety of ways.

Qualifications and Curriculum Development Agency (QCDA)

83 Piccadilly, London W1J 8QA
Tel: 0300 303 3011
www.qcda.gov.uk

The QCDA website covers every aspect of 14 to 19
education, including the Diploma in Hair and Beauty
Studies.

Scottish Qualifications Authority (SQA)

The Optima Building, 58 Robertson Street, Glasgow
G2 8DQ
Tel: 0845 279 1000
www.sqa.org.uk

SQA has broad responsibility for qualifications below
degree level in Scotland. The website covers a range of
qualifications including SVQs.

UCAS

Rosehill, New Barn Lane, Cheltenham GL52 3LZ
Tel: 01242 222444
www.ucas.ac.uk

UCAS processes more than two million applications for full-time undergraduate courses every year and can help you find the right higher education course.

Vocational Training Charitable Trust (VTCT)
Third Floor, Eastleigh House, Upper Market Street, Eastleigh SO50 9FD
Tel: 023 8068 4500
www.vtct.org.uk

VTCT is the government-approved specialist awarding body for the hairdressing and beauty sector. It has provided internationally recognised qualifications for over 40 years and offers a range of qualifications in hairdressing and barbering.

PERIODICALS

The list below is far from exhaustive but it includes titles widely read in the industry.

Black Beauty and Hair
www.blackbeautyandhair.com

Published every two months by Hawker Consumer Publications Ltd, this is widely acknowledged as a leading magazine on black hair and beauty. Regular features include product reviews, celebrity interviews and hair and beauty advice pages. The target readership is the 18- to 34-year-old age range.

Habia News magazine
www.habia.org

Habia News is published several times a year and is the leading source of information on education and training in the hair and beauty sector. It is free to all Habia members and you can find back issues online.

Hair
IPC Media

This glossy monthly magazine is aimed primarily at 14- to 24-year-olds. It includes tips and advice from top hairdressers, news about the latest products on the market and step-by-step guides to achieving the perfect look.

Hair Ideas
www.loveyourhair.com

This handbag-sized monthly magazine, published by Origin Publishing, is broadly aimed at a 14- to 30-year-old audience. Like its sister magazine, *Your Hair*, it aims to inspire readers through everything from celebrity features to quick tips and step-by-step guides.

Hairdressers Journal International
www.hji.co.uk

The magazine brings the latest fashions, product information, event coverage, industry news and career opportunities to its readers every week. From students through to experienced stylists, HJ is all about inspiring today's hairdresser. The interactive website includes a huge image gallery and online hairdressing community.

BOOKS

Habia produces a broad range of publications, some of which are geared to trainees. You might find these two of interest.

Illustrated Hairdressing Dictionary by Jane Hiscock, Nicci Moorman and Leah Palmer (ref. BK-142, £16.99), an easy-to-use dictionary designed especially for hairdressing students.

Student Handbook

Every year, Habia produces a student handbook, which is a mine of information on everything from career paths to protecting your health. You can download a copy from the Habia Member Schools section of the website (www. habia.org).

CHAPTER 14
JARGON BUSTERS

Bouffant

The bouffant is a hairstyle in which the hair is piled high on top of the head, with tendrils hanging down at the sides. It was very popular in the early to mid 1960s, when women used large amounts of hairspray to keep the style in place.

Chemical relaxing

Chemical relaxing involves applying chemicals to curly or wavy hair to straighten it. Like perming (permanent waving), it changes the structure of the hair, but the opposite way round: perming adds waves or curls whereas chemical relaxing removes them.

Fingerwaving

Fingerwaving is the art of moulding damp hair into 'S' shapes using only fingers, comb, setting lotion and hairpins. The hair dries into waves without heat being applied.

Five point cut

This short, precisely cut hairstyle is still copied by hairdressers around the world. Created by Vidal Sassoon, it is an adapted version of the classic bob hairstyle.

Lacquered

Lacquered hair was heavily hairsprayed to keep the style in place.

Long hairdressing

Long hairdressing is the art of styling and arranging long hair in either an upswept style or down. It can involve a range of techniques, including adding extra hair and ornamentation.